Hungry For Diets
Why Diets Don't Work

Your No-Diet Book

Jesse CRAIGNOU

Hungry for Diets
Everything you've always wanted to know about diets… and yet were never told !

Jesse CRAIGNOU

About my writing

Coming from a multinational multicultural family I learnt many languages and to deal with many cultures…
This has shown me the importance of words and communication.

Words are sweet water to my lips…
For lack of a better word I'll make up my own if I have to… if it serves the purpose of my writing… words are all yet sometimes words are not enough…

From the minute I could write I wrote… on everything and anything I could fin to write on… I wrote I wrote I wrote… and I haven't stopped writing yet…
My first memory of writing was at home writing my name on my little blackboard… My father came to correct it… and writing was on for me from that moment on…

There was a time poetry belonged in popular culture before it was held hostage by the elite…
In many respects and ways I have long felt I belong in those days…
People quoted and cited lines from poems as people today sing along the streets…
And words were their music…

A couple of years ago one of my students presented a piece of his work about Louise BENNETT -the first Jamaican woman poet- and he got me thinking on how I wish I could go back to the dawn of writing… to be the first person ever to write the first book in his language… the first fiction…
Or even… Bulgarian born Elias CANETTI who, from wanting so much to understand the private thoughts his parents shared in German, went on to become one of the greatest German writers of his time and beyond… because with writing comes history… and come stories… and communication…

My main interests belong in life, people and nature.
People usually don't see the surrealistic aspects of their life… when I do…

Most of my endeavours are about communication… and my writings are very oral in fact… they are meant to be heard and said more than read… even if one should indeed enjoy reading them… whether books, texts, poems or songs they would easily find their way to the radio or stage… and I have recorded a few that I offer for sale now…

I also write for business and communication as well as for children… in a style that blends fact and fiction as well as poetry and prose… writing about people for people…

Most of my books come in French and in English.

#benefit, #cost, #diet, #disorder, #doctor, #eat, #food, #guide, #heal, #health, #junk, #nutrition, #recipe, #sport, #walk, #weight,

Hungry for Diets
Everything you've always wanted to know about diets… and yet were never told !

Jesse CRAIGNOU

In **Hunger For Diets** I revisit the work of my life… of my study of food and its effects and consequences on the body… on our metabolism…

Not one doctor… not one specialist… not one study… has ever lasted as long as my study !

#benefit, #cost, #diet, #disorder, #doctor, #eat, #food, #guide, #heal, #health, #junk, #nutrition, #recipe, #sport, #walk, #weight,

Hungry for Diets
Everything you've always wanted to know about diets… and yet were never told !

Jesse CRAIGNOU

About my writing

Thank you

Words
Books
Audio books
PodCasts

#benefit, #cost, #diet, #disorder, #doctor, #eat, #food, #guide, #heal, #health, #junk, #nutrition, #recipe, #sport, #walk, #weight,

Hungry for Diets
Everything you've always wanted to know about diets… and yet were never told !

Jesse CRAIGNOU

Training & Coaching

Translating

Paris Guide

#benefit, #cost, #diet, #disorder, #doctor, #eat, #food, #guide, #heal, #health, #junk, #nutrition, #recipe, #sport, #walk, #weight,

page 5 of 87

Jesse CRAIGNOU

One diet here today one diet gone tomorrow…
All diets work… while you're on that diet…
All successful diet books have been written by people in wonderful shape… who most of the time have never even put their diet to the test… but who didn't think twice about making their fortune on the fat of their readers… and those who have tested it based their miracle recipe on the fact that it worked for them –i.e. 1 person !-
They describe a wonderful world in which we all hold the solution within ourselves… and so much for the better…
So then why are so many people overweight ? You may ask…

It is estimated in our industrialised countries, that at least 60 % of people are overweight, most of them obese or obese-to-be… to become and stay obese…
95 % of the people who go on a diet fail… recalls doctor and cardiologist Dr Saldmann… and I would add end up stalked by their diets !

The market for diets is one of the profitable ones in the world ! And with 100s of millions of overweight people in the world diet evangelists can have their cake and eat it…
Let's go and see what results diets get…

One man's meat is another man's poison…

What's your diet ?
Not one doctor or nutritionist has ever asked me what I ate… nor even followed up what they recommended… as it is few of them ask us what caused our ailments…
We are going to look at all the options and the questions doctors, paramedics and health professionals never ask us –or themselves- !

In 2014, I eat 3 times less bread and 5 times less potatoes than 40 years ago… all the best of 50 years of brainwashing from the moment the medical profession and diet evangelists banned them from our tables… only to eventually rehab them ! A battle so hard to fight that they had to convince us with painstaking and lengthy efforts of convincing us that they were not bad for our weight… and even good for our health !

The worst is one can be in perfect health without ever eating healthy food !

Let's take a good look at the effects and results of diets over the long run…
Doctors and nutritionists only look at us over a comparatively short spell…

#benefit, #cost, #diet, #disorder, #doctor, #eat, #food, #guide, #heal, #health, #junk, #nutrition, #recipe, #sport, #walk, #weight,

Hungry for Diets
Everything you've always wanted to know about diets… and yet were never told !

Jesse CRAIGNOU

Who eats what ?
Who needs a diet ? Which diet(s) really give long term results ?
What are bad eating habits ?

Nobody has ever wanted nor enjoyed being overweight… and if, as a young man, I used to think that anybody was overweight or obese was because they overate or didn't take care of their shape, I realised all along my life and that of thousands of people I have met that it wasn't the case… far from it… I was totally wrong…

Hungry for Diets
Everything you've always wanted to know about diets… and yet were never told !

Old habits die hard… and so do old clichés…

No matter how obvious this is… we are constantly told and retold the same old wives' tales and recipes…
The diet prophets don't give in easily…

I am offering to compare and share experiences and conclusions… resting on the examples of reasonable eaters… like me…

All the diets we are proffered work… for some time… over the short run… on people who have the worst eating habits and/or overeat…
We are never told about people who have weight problems but don't overeat or have eating disorders…

If it were enough to cut down on food and exercise a little the whole world would be slim… and easily too… we wouldn't need all those malevolent doctors, nutritionists and other fitness centres and training apparatuses… who only make us suffer !

And if there were one diet that worked one would serve all !

#benefit, #cost, #diet, #disorder, #doctor, #eat, #food, #guide, #heal, #health, #junk, #nutrition, #recipe, #sport, #walk, #weight,

page 8 of 87

Jesse CRAIGNOU

Diet Victim – In the Beginning was the Fat

I have been on every diet ! Every single one !
My family has been on all of them too… each and everyone of us on each and everyone one of them…
We took out, changed, put in, included, swapped, traded, … all to no avail !

I will always remember my mother, forever overweight, on one diet or another… again and again… she would exercise in the bedroom every morning for 20 minutes… while leading a mother and a professional lifestyles all the while… managing farms then restaurants… both fields which require excellent health and provide lots of healthy exercise… never to see the benefits of all her good work and endless efforts… nothing, I tell you, not the slightest difference at the end of the day…

Among all the members of my family we compile more diet experience than all the nutritionists, dieticians, and doctors in the world… still no one ever asked us… and no one ever listened to us… if we were fat it was because we ate like horses and were lazy bums !
All my life has been nothing but a never-ending relentless fight against overweight… without ever giving up… even for one meal… even in times of despair…
I spent my whole life chasing salt, sugar, fat, oils, starch, laziness… chasing both food and life… only to find that all those ingredients have now been rehabbed and are praised for the good they do to our body and metabolism… and that everything we were told all along was wrong all along… the gurus and the times had changed… and diets too… and I came out every time with a feeling of irrevocable injustice that I would forever remain the prisoner of my ill-fated body…

No diet has ever worked in the long run… no diet has ever worked in the mid run… I only ended wondering whether all those efforts were worth the pain of no gain… my only gain was weight…

Shocking !
To be told again and again every time I see a doctor not to eat fat, fried, starchy foods, desserts, eating between meals, binging, sugar and alcohol… in a word everything I don't eat !
I was nearing avoiding all food…
My religion challenged anorexia…

No one had ever asked me what I ate… or didn't eat… and when I tried to tell them no one listened…

#benefit, #cost, #diet, #disorder, #doctor, #eat, #food, #guide, #heal, #health, #junk, #nutrition, #recipe, #sport, #walk, #weight,

Jesse CRAIGNOU

What kind of doctors are those ? Who doesn't even listen to his patients…

And when they did listen they started sending me on a guilt trip… '*That's what you all say… yet the truth is you're eating too much of all this !*'
First, I am not the others… second, why would I go and seek help to lose weight if I stuffed my face… and not one of them has ever come to check my fridge…
Need I say that not one of them has ever made me lose any weight… except Montignac… who is not a doctor !
All they ever did was blame me… lie to me and listen to no one but themselves…

As a teenager I had a friend who was grossly overweight… and her brother who was rather good-looking had found nothing better than nickname her Fattie… and so did all the kids at college… she used to skip meals and starve herself to lose weight… all to no avail… while trying to keep that Couldn't-care-less' smile on her face… but deep down she knew she was lost…
I sympathised secretly with our Fattie… knowing only too well what she was going through… although at her age only 2 thirds of her size and comparatively slim…
The 70s cultivated slimness and the 80s sculpted everyone's body… but Fattie exhibited her Beth Ditto looks… a long time before her days…

My two sisters hardly ever ate anything when they were little and one of them had been nicknamed Toothpick as a baby in the maternity ward… being the tiniest baby they had ever seen… the same sister who, aged 42, after years and years of intensive sport and a severely monitored diet peaked at 102 kilos for 1,5 meter in height… already in the past she had been on a Slim Fast diet which made her put on 40 kilos…

My other sister and brother have always been chubby… never did any sports and always ate as much as they could… and pleased…
Most of the career sports people reach 40 with weight in excess…

A famous doctor running her own TV show from the beginning of the 80s when she had a figure any model who have dreamt of…
30 years later, she is 4 times her young size and yet continues preaching health through hygiene and careful eating and dieting… without the slightest hint of a doubt…

I have seen obese children whose parents watch the diet and exercise as though their life depended on it… blaming, accusing, their offspring to go and eat behind their backs… worse, I have seen people track the small crumb, the calories, the grams, the kilos… with an unbridled unrivalled obsession without ever finding grace

#benefit, #cost, #diet, #disorder, #doctor, #eat, #food, #guide, #heal, #health, #junk, #nutrition, #recipe, #sport, #walk, #weight,

in the face of fat… or, worse still, those who had to go on a diet while the verged on skin and bones…

I'm 22 and I have lost almost 30 kilos swimming… I have an athlete's body and am so light I feel like I'm going to take off on the first gush of wind… my doctor cannot believe it… he doesn't believe me… '*So you've been on that diet at last*' he grunts happily… '*No doctor, I have not been on that diet, I've been swimming*'… he calls in his secretary to ask her to remind him he should send his overweight patients to the swimming pool…
For years I keep my weight down and seem free from all dietary expectations…

I'm 35 and I've lost 20 kilos thanks to Montignac, phase 2, without the slightest effort nor diet to my name… I have lost so much weight people who know me daren't ask me how I am for fearing I have a severe major ailment… I feel better than I have ever felt…
I keep my weight down until my late forties…

I'm 50 and neither Montignac nor sports nor diet can do anything for me…
I subscribed for one year at the swimming pool where I go almost everyday… I have a rower at home I use to exercise 20 minutes a day… but my body refuses to know… to answer my pleas… only one result… my back lies in total tatters…

I have practiced sports incessantly ever since childhood… and have been on diets ever since early childhood… without anything to show for it…

My last visit to my cardiologist I had clocked up another 4 kilos ! After weeks of having lived –survived- on salads… I ate even less and had noticed I was 'eliminating' more… and rightly thought I had 'lost' weight… in the summer I literally live on gazpacho… damned metabolism !

Beyond disappointment and inconvenience… there is the cost !
Overweight people have more health problems and have to take more medicine – often causing more trouble with side effects-… overweight people need to buy more clothes… an extra cost not everybody can afford…

I have seen my parents and their parents and relatives spend their life on diets through and through… some of them eventually giving their body up to plastic surgery… the only way out…
A few of those brothers and sisters of mine who have never been on a diet… show no difference in terms of size or weight… as well all the sports freaks…

#benefit, #cost, #diet, #disorder, #doctor, #eat, #food, #guide, #heal, #health, #junk, #nutrition, #recipe, #sport, #walk, #weight,

page 11 of 87

Hungry for Diets
Everything you've always wanted to know about diets… and yet were never told !

Jesse CRAIGNOU

In a family of 2 boys and 2 girls… one of my sisters and I have devoted our lives to sports and dieting… the other two did not… and well are all overweight today…

Nobody has ever looked into the reason for my excess weight… food, eating habits, osteopathy, genetics, or other…
All the diets, all the types of food, all the sports have led to the same results… whatever I do…
I have been massaged, have taken dietary supplements, all the potions, all the hunger reducers, all the fat burners, all the detoxifiers… and anything else that came my way or was offered or proffered to me… and of course everything the doctors ordered… nothing I tell you… nothing has made the slightest difference !
Fat burners and detoxifiers made me hungry… and fed me cravings I had never known before them… I wouldn't recommend fat burners anyway as the brain is made up of fat… it is not sure whether they actually affect the brain… one thing is sure… when I was on fat burners I kept having those terrible headaches… I didn't have without them… to be taken under supervision and with the utmost care… if you ask me…

All I could do was helplessly watch those kilos pile up on my body… without my being able to do anything about it… nobody understands… nobody can explain this assault on my body… I remain the prisoner of a heartless body that behaves as it pleases…

Difficult to imagine that the microscopic cell that is a spermatozoid may evolve to weigh anything up to 500 kilos (half a ton !) for the most extreme cases… and for some animals tons and tons…

#benefit, #cost, #diet, #disorder, #doctor, #eat, #food, #guide, #heal, #health, #junk, #nutrition, #recipe, #sport, #walk, #weight,

Jesse CRAIGNOU

To your Health !

For the best part of the past 100 years we have been offered diets, medicines, lotions and magic potions, if one worked we would all know it… and would walk over anybody's body to get it ! If one had worked the fortune of the discoverer would be made… and we would all live on a planet of top models… and all of the medical field would be the first to be slim…

The news would make headline news all over the world… unless all those dietpreneurs have no better wish than keep us in the dark… and in the fat… so as to sell us more of their stuff ?

Most of the honest and earnest dietpreneurs today join the fat of the troop… and admit to not having the solution to get rid of excess weight… still they're all still in the game…

Many even fend against colleagues… directly or via the media… and/or patients only to prove –by fair means or foul- that they are right when all the evidence is against them… they only listen to their ego…

Most of us have to reckon rather than reconcile with the fact that come 40 and up to 60 we're in for an unwanted weight gain… whatever our metabolism or genetics may be to start with…

Most of us start at 30 even… mothers will know what I'm talking about… and all that nature is putting on hold for a while… but only for a while… if we go for sports… and again most sports people and all those stars who have made us dream with their looks… start bucking under their weight with age… which leaves much to be desired…

A 70s pop foursome featuring 2 female vocalists… both slim although one 'rounder'… 40 years later the fleshier of the 2 is thin as a rake… and the slimmer has gone the other way…

All the same British (Dr Lesley Regan) and American studies show that the effects and properties of medicine, dietary supplements, food (whether organic or not), probiotics, pesticides, etc… have, within reasonable measures, no effect… at the worst neither is more noxious nor beneficial on the body… as the metabolism rejects most of them in its great wisdom… after retaining whatever is beneficial for the body… whereas the placebo and/or nocebo effects and any other psychosomatic approaches work anytime !

Again in the UK, professor Susan Jebb studied the effect of fat and sugar over a 10 year period… to conclude that reducing and/or withdrawing sugar and fat from food has virtually no effect on the weight or health…

#benefit, #cost, #diet, #disorder, #doctor, #eat, #food, #guide, #heal, #health, #junk, #nutrition, #recipe, #sport, #walk, #weight,

However the body transforms the fat into sugar… that in turn transforms into fat that turns into sugar… that turns into fat… and again into sugar… in turns ad libitum…

The body obviously has its reasons… which reason ignores… the mystery gets more mysterious… as we eat…

All the studies tend to prove that excess weight goes against good health… but what is health actually ? All the data on excess weight are elastic and iffy at best… many defy the laws of health and nobody seems to be interested in metabolism… which would probably have both interesting and relevant information to teach us…

There are places in our world where ethnic groups seem to escape excess weight… the same goes for most underdeveloped or developing countries… where obesity is so rare that is adulated and worshipped… strange world…

At the dawn of mankind, and thus over millennia, man took his food wherever he found it or whatever ate he liked when and where food was plentiful… without any further question as to the benefits of food on his body… and nobody could tell that resulted in any effect either on his body… or the 'natural' size…

The Inuit
While we are constantly rehashed the benefits of a well balanced diet, the Inuit have lived on meat and fat alone ever since they came into existence…

North and South American (Native) Indians
Just like the Inuit North and South American Indian populations rely mostly on meat for their diet…

The Samba in Mauritania
Again just like the Inuit and American Indians they rely mostly on meat (fish) for their food supply…

The Chinese and Asians
The Chinese and Far East Asians have always eaten fat and sweet food… and yet have remained slim all along… with the exception of the Japanese… who, with a similar diet, also 'underfeed' themselves… the average Japanese leaves the table while still hungry… as it is in their culture…
They are also usually in better health than Europeans and Americans… and hardly ever take medicine…
Health is ideology –as well as nutritional and medical terrorism- pure speculation… and one man's poison is another man's meat… while is some cultures healthy means

Jesse CRAIGNOU

slim, lean and thin in other cultures healthy is big and fat… yet, at the end of the day, no one nowhere lives better nor older than the others…

We cannot help but notice while studying all the nutritional modes… as I have always done rather than mechanically repeat hearsay or any aberration issue by the medical and paramedical profession… and see that the whole concept of health and healthy eating is begging to be revisited… and that's exactly what I'm calling for in this very book…

In my youth eating fish, fruit and vegetable was the lot of poor people… as those foods were much cheaper than meat… but today they are as expensive if not more…

At closer inspection eating more fruit or vegetables is no more than a mere political roll call for sponsoring an agriculture they have long and hard worked to kill… clearly none of this nonsense has anything to do with nutritional logic !

Neither the Inuit nor the American Indians… nor even the Samba have ever heard of the balanced diets, which are recommended to the white man for his health… and neither have all the other people of all the deserts and all the jungles in the world…
We are told people in cold countries eat more than other people to face the low temperatures… yet people in warm and hot countries often eat richer foods offering more calories and fat and sugar all thrown in…
All along my life and rich experience of eating and meeting people from all over the world… as well as living in different countries… coming from a family of mixed origins and cultures myself… I have noticed people all over the world are relatively similar when it comes to size and weight… regardless of what they may eat…
It would take someone who has never left home… never met anyone… never watched television to believe otherwise… and not to know this…

Many times swimming champion Florent M confesses to loving junk food and eating nothing else… almost to the point of advertising it… and yet he sports a dream body… and enjoys great health…

Vegetarians and vegans eat more than meat eaters… they also eat less and more often… as meat diets offer richer nutrients that require a longer digestion time… whereas vegetarian and vegan diets are made up of nutrients more challenging to digest for man (gasses)… but digesting those nutrients is also faster and imposes more meals every day… and a more developed digestive track…

In their various countries and cultures people will eat different things in different proportions… yet they all face the same challenge… there are rarely less fat people in one country than in another… and yet all the diet and nutrition specialists give

#benefit, #cost, #diet, #disorder, #doctor, #eat, #food, #guide, #heal, #health, #junk, #nutrition, #recipe, #sport, #walk, #weight,

them the same diets… with the same results… this should give any doctor or paramedic food for thought…

It seems that whatever we may eat the result is the same in the long run… or the difference barely significant… whether obscure or hypothetical… diets when they claim to work… only work as long as the dieter is on that diet…

#benefit, #cost, #diet, #disorder, #doctor, #eat, #food, #guide, #heal, #health, #junk, #nutrition, #recipe, #sport, #walk, #weight,

page 16 of 87

Jesse CRAIGNOU

Overweight, obesity

'*With the event of the automobile civilisation, man has started to run…*'
Régis DEBRÉ

Some people will always see themselves as overweight… and will compulsively diet… to the point of bulimia or anorexia nervosa… or any other suchlike eating aberration and disorder… as more commonly found in women… while others will always see themselves as too skinny… whereas the two parties may be of the same size !

Their vision is perverted… disrupted in a way that doesn't reflect their true physiognomy… right next to them top models ferociously track down the slightest – and lightest- unwanted gram of flesh…

We are not all equal in the weight war…
Some will put on a lot of weight without eating hardly anything… while others will lose little at the expense of great efforts… or will shed weight without asking for it or eating any the less than before…
Some will lose weight when they're anxious or depressed… while others will gain weight when they're anxious or depressed… without changing anything to their diets…

So then where does obesity start ?
I would say that overweight starts when the individual in question sees him/herself as such… or society sees him/her as such… whichever way is wrong… yet applies in any case as I'm sure we have all noticed…

For some it is a question of beauty… and being skinny or slim promotes ugliness… and for those obesity is beauty…

The question is… when health is really at stake…

The first question that needs be asked is '*What kind of fat are you ?*'
There is more than one kind of fat !
Does your fat come from overeating or aberrant eating pattern, lack of exercise, genetics, metabolic laziness or disorder, thyroid disorder, oedema, medicinal side effects, …

#benefit, #cost, #diet, #disorder, #doctor, #eat, #food, #guide, #heal, #health, #junk, #nutrition, #recipe, #sport, #walk, #weight,

Jesse CRAIGNOU

Raiders of the Lost Fat

Diets

The French National Food & Health Environment & Work Agency (ANSES) published back in November 2010 an expert's report on the assessment of risks linked to dieting.

'Diets, done without recommendation nor a specialist's follow-up are very widespread among the public through the channels of distribution and the Internet present health hazards ranging from the smallest to the worst'… as estimated by the ANSES.
The report shows the noxious effects on the metabolism, and particularly on the bones, the heart, and the kidneys, as much as on the psychological side, especially in the event of the development of bad eating habits…

Why do diets make people fat ?
An estimated 80-95 % of people lose weight within 5 years (the Yoyo Effect)
The reason ?
The hypercontrol of food and mental that most diets impose on the dieters…

Even if the analysis of eating behaviour reveals a severe complexity (genetics, psychological, socio-environmental, and psycho-emotional factors), studies show today there is a definite interaction between emotions and eating behaviour…
The control of eating habits is done by mechanisms most of which are unconscious…

We will look here at potential dieters who have reasonable and non-outrageous eating habits…

#benefit, #cost, #diet, #disorder, #doctor, #eat, #food, #guide, #heal, #health, #junk, #nutrition, #recipe, #sport, #walk, #weight,

page 18 of 87

Jesse CRAIGNOU

Diets resurface at least once a year… just like the snake Apophis coming back to warm himself under the rays of Ra, to whom he almost lost its skin…

No diet has ever given proof of being concretely efficient in the long run !
It's a shame… scandalous… all the experts' conclusions go that way…

The first inconvenience of a diet is that it comes as the life-long sentence without any hope of appeal voiced as though by an unsympathetic Torquemada…
This is where we find the cause of an announced failure…
The unavowed cause of failures is that not one of those diets works… no matter how hard you try and work at it…

Of course when starting a diet everybody loses weight at the speed of light… kilos just seem to melt away like ice in the sun… and the hope of redemption seems to rise on the horizon line…
But the pangs of reality (too) soon take over and soon shed the light on the sad realisation of the fate of the bon viveur…

We know now, thanks to constant scientific progress, so much more about our metabolism… and that progress progresses every year… and year after year…
All the offers of diets can only liken themselves to those of the climate future of the planet… escalating to the craziest theories… so much is our arrogance to believe we know best and will win every time…
It is obvious that we still know so little… if anything at all… of who or what will bring the answer to this cheeky question…
Life and nature show us everyday that our forecasts like yesterday's hypotheses are utterly wrong ! And at best the truth is a far cry from the goal posts…

Diets aiming at lowering our cholesterol and fat have only been met with less than little success so far… as it is not what we eat that matters anyway… except maybe in the event of diabetes and hyperglycemia, outside aberrant eating behaviours… nothing controls cholesterol in the body as it is the body that produces 90 % of its own cholesterol… and fortunately so too… as the body needs cholesterol to fill the breaks and splits in our aging breaking veins ! Going against this natural process may even prove hazardous in the mid to long run…
And yet doctors and medical experts as well as nutritionists don't give up… and continue preaching it is necessary to reduce fat intake… even to those who never take any !
The only real treatment will be that which manages the cholesterol production… if the body should fail… so long as that production doesn't become invasive and blocks the veins and arteries… to the point of preventing blood circulation…

#benefit, #cost, #diet, #disorder, #doctor, #eat, #food, #guide, #heal, #health, #junk, #nutrition, #recipe, #sport, #walk, #weight,

Jesse CRAIGNOU

Archaeologists are now finding while studying mummies found everywhere in the world that all our forefathers 'suffered' from cholesterol and atherosclerosis… thus it is useless for doctors to blame their patients for their bad eating habits… and their lack of physical exercise…

One of my friends has just been to see his dietician…to lose a few kilos…

At 42 he has always had an intense and regular physical activity practising sports both to keep fit and for pleasure several times a week… but he doesn't accept that buoy settling around his waist…

His nutritionist immediately asks him to keep away from… everything they all tell us to keep away from… in cases like his… but we all know that…

Honestly who needs to go and see a nutritionist to be told to keep away from fat and sugar… and exercise ? We all know that !

Strangely I have never seen an old nutritionist… they all seem to come young…

That or their career is short-lived…

The only rare chosen few who survive end up working in hospitals…

Strange in a world where so many people would need them… and in growing numbers too !

The same friend who was telling me the other day that, having taken up sports again, he has shed 7 kilos in 6 months… he proudly announces he has come down to 77 kilos (I weighed 72 kilos at that age for 5 cm shorter than he is)…

Not one of those diets that ask the dieter to cut down, avoid, change, or a remix of their food is ever successful !

They all leave an aftertaste of hunger for food and cravings… leaving the dieter very frustrated… the minute we're ask to cut anything out of our staple diet we want more of it…

All those diets soon meet their limits and, what with the drastic limits they impose, put us off almost immediately… as we all know…

And what's worse… the more we deprive our body of something the more our body stocks it… it's a natural process…

Even liposuction only brings temporary local relief as we soon see fat reappear… elsewhere on the body… if not in the same place… what is now called 'deep fat' !

If losing weight were down to eating a little less or doing exercise… it would be so simple and easy…

How are we supposed to feel when we've tried everything under the sun… and that against all odds and all we can see is… our body grow and expand and weigh down on us… and weigh you down ? That we're under the impression from waking up that our body has managed to put on weight during our sleep… behind our back ?

#benefit, #cost, #diet, #disorder, #doctor, #eat, #food, #guide, #heal, #health, #junk, #nutrition, #recipe, #sport, #walk, #weight,

Jesse CRAIGNOU

Diets and their Pitfalls

Man was never made to go on diets…

Let's look at **diets** again…

What are diets and balanced diets really worth ?
Let's face it… most diets are about depriving us of one thing or another… or others… and their top of the charts are sugar and fat, added –or rather withdrawn from- to that starch… and they promote reengineering eating and exercise… which takes us back to the dawn of dieting… with the results we know…

All the screen stars –whether small or big silver screen, who have ever been overweight- have written their book promoting their miracle diet… with a high return on investment as those books always sell well… even if we often meet those same stars in the mid to long run having regained their excess weight… miracle diets often hiding the desperate secret of a plastic surgery operation…

There are books from doctors and nutritionists, gurus, freaks, those of before and those of after…

#benefit, #cost, #diet, #disorder, #doctor, #eat, #food, #guide, #heal, #health, #junk, #nutrition, #recipe, #sport, #walk, #weight,

page 21 of 87

Jesse CRAIGNOU

Let's check them one after the other with all the evidence of the most popular ones...

For mothers, **the after baby diet**...
Nothing new here : moderation, exercise and balance... without ever telling the dieting mother that the body is supposed to go back to what it was... before the pregnancy... naturally... and there are mothers who even lose weight after the baby is born... to go down to a lighter body than the one they had before the pregnancy... then again being a mother is quite an exercise as it is !

The Karl Lagerfeld diet
Moderation and balance.

The Véronique Genest diet
Low calorie diet.

The Sonia Dubois' diet
Moderation and balance. Difficult.
The famous journalist hasn't kept the benefits of her diet though...

Sulitzer's diet
Balanced diet. Fibres.

The Stars' diet
Moderation and balance. Difficult.

Dr Benchetrit's diet
Nothing new: Moderation and balance.

Dr Cohen's diet
Reengineering eating habits.

Dr Dukan diet
Proteins. Bashed because can induce major health problems... Dr Dukan has been taken to court many times by both clients and colleagues...

Dr Siegal's diet
Too low in fibres.
May lead to bowel trouble.

The Low Calorie diet
Many versions.
#benefit, #cost, #diet, #disorder, #doctor, #eat, #food, #guide, #heal, #health, #junk, #nutrition, #recipe, #sport, #walk, #weight,

Low in sugar and calories.
Should prove well balanced but a job to keep on.

Jenny Craig's diet
Reengineering eating habits.
Includes a telephone follow-up (once a week) by a "consultant", in actual fact a would-be dietician… trained on the approach !

The Soup diet
Low calorie. The weight is soon back on.

The Zone aka Dr Sears's diet
Low in sugar. Moderation and balance.

Weight Watchers' diet
Moderation and balance. Everything is limited. Pleasant and game-like synergy… positive.

The High Protein and Substitutes' diet
High in proteins and low in calories.
Dieters lose weight fast but… also put it back on fast. …

Dr Atkins's diet
No sugar, rich fat.
To ban… especially for those who do a lot of exercise… may lead to a lot of health troubles.

The Blood Group diet
Dieting recommendations as per your blood group.
Has become very rare… and doesn't seem to have much to show in the line of results…

The Moon Phase diet
Eating in phase with the moon. Freakish…

The Instinctive diet
Eat what you want… whenever you want… as per what your body leads you to eat…

The Neanderthal diet
Eating like our forefathers… I will let you imagine what hell it must be to run out of mammoth steak or roast… once you've found one !

#benefit, #cost, #diet, #disorder, #doctor, #eat, #food, #guide, #heal, #health, #junk, #nutrition, #recipe, #sport, #walk, #weight,

Jesse CRAIGNOU

The Top Model diet
Eat only steamed green beans and brown rice… not the best promoter of a balanced diet but surely easy enough if boring… most people don't last a week…

The Yin and Yang diet
Balance and control.

The Hollywood or Fruit diet
Unbalanced and monotonous. Bad for the digestive track.

The Low-Carb diet
Low in sugar.
Monotonous in the mid to long run.

The Mayo diet
Low in calories and unbalanced.

The Miami diet
Low in calories and unbalanced.

The Scarsdale diet
Low in calories and sugar.

The Chrono diet
Chrononutrition. Low in calories.

The Antoine diet
The Shelton diet
The Montignac diet
Disassociated and low in calories.
The **disassociated food** diet, with their digestive and assimilative approach, offers a logical logistics… This diet promotes a better digestion and rests the metabolism while most toxins are naturally eliminated… enabling an enhanced operation of both the metabolism and body…

The IG diet
Low in sugar.

The Basic Acids diet
Detox and low in acids.

#benefit, #cost, #diet, #disorder, #doctor, #eat, #food, #guide, #heal, #health, #junk, #nutrition, #recipe, #sport, #walk, #weight,

Hungry for Diets
Everything you've always wanted to know about diets… and yet were never told !

Jesse CRAIGNOU

The Hypnosis diet
To re-educate eating habits.
For the victims of nutritional aberrations.

The Detox diet
Spring cleaning the metabolism.

The Medium Fat diet
Low in calories and sugar. Mediterranean.

The Okinawa diet
Low in calories and sugar.
Fish instead of meat and lots of vegetables.
Remember that the Japanese also undereat.

The Zermati diet
Constraints and re-education.

The Slim-Data diet
Low in sugar.

Dr Fricker's diet
Low in calories and sugar while re-educating eating habits. Highly demanding.

The Astronaut's diet
Low in calories and sugar while re-educating eating habits. Underfeeding.

The Gordon diet
Dieting and underfeeding.

The Messini diet
Low in calories and sugar while re-educating eating habits. Underfeeding.

The PSMF diet
Low in calories and sugar while re-educating eating habits. Underfeeding and low in proteins.

The Razzoli diet
Low in calories.

The Cold diet
Bla bla bla…

#benefit, #cost, #diet, #disorder, #doctor, #eat, #food, #guide, #heal, #health, #junk, #nutrition, #recipe, #sport, #walk, #weight,

Jesse CRAIGNOU

The Liquid diet
Mostly vegetable and dietary supplements mix… blended and liquidised… found to be lethal to dieters, who tended to lose their teeth after a wile…

High in proteins diets seem to lower –at least for a period- the water retention and thus promote weight loss… without, however, providing a long term benefit or solution…

No diet works over the long term… once the benefits –when there are any at all- have gone… even while remaining on that diet the body goes back to its (over)weight as it adapts itself… all the nutrition specialists and doctors will eventually admit to that… worse still is the Yoyo Effect… which causes major damage to the body and metabolism…
No matter which diet we go for and how many times we change… we lose weight every time… and every time our body adjusts itself… until the next diet…

All sorts of diets are on offer… Even the richest in fat !

The Paleo diet promotes eating fat in excess… and it gets results in weight loss or no weight gain… eating fat, especially in the morning, would promote a better metabolisation of the food… by reducing the hunger feeling and the cravings… and thus making the dieter eat less… and lose weight… who knows ?
The Americans have pushed to such extreme and sectarian –while depriving- diets that they now have to take massive doses of dietary supplements… ranging from the most beneficial to the freakiest… at the expense of their health…

Just as cosmetics, which claim to maintain that youthful look on your face, although generally breaking the rules of legal practice, bring no results in actual facts… apart from boosting individual vanity… and lightening the dieter's wallet…

The diet or weight reducing product beneficial over the long term is yet to come !

#benefit, #cost, #diet, #disorder, #doctor, #eat, #food, #guide, #heal, #health, #junk, #nutrition, #recipe, #sport, #walk, #weight,

Jesse CRAIGNOU

American study on 4 diets... (Suppression of fat, sugar, starch, ...)

An American diet study on 811 overweight dieters over a period of 2 years…

Researchers recruited 811 overweight adults and asked them to go on 1 of 4 diets… 2 of which promoted low calories with 2 diets reducing by 20 % the fat intake and 2 diets promoting reducing of 40 % of fat intake… the carbon calories varied from 35 to 65 %... the proteins make up as much as 15 to 25 % of calories…

The 4 diets met the principles of cardiac health, which imposes to consume less than 8 % of calories coming from saturated animal fat likely to bring on clots in the arteries, to eat vegetables, fruit and whole flour, and to eat at least 20 grams of fibres every day…

The 4 diets rested on the precepts of DASH (Dietary Approaches to Stop Hypertension) and not on diets such as the Dr Atkins' or South Beach Diets…
The participants have been requested to take part in regular individual or group sessions and to keep a diary on the food they ate… each participant has been assigned a target reduction of 750 calories on their daily intake… none of them is supposed to consume less than 1,200 calories daily…
The exercise objectives remained on average at about 90 minutes of moderate exercise weekly…

The researchers' job was to observe how the diets influenced the weight loss in order not to tamper with the results…

The results were published in the New England Journal of Medicine as follows :

In 6 months the participants lost on average 13 pounds… whichever diet they were on.

After 2 years they remained on an average of 13 pounds and had lost 1 to 3 inches in waist, whichever diet they were on…

The participants had improved their cardiac risk factor, including a rise in HDL (good) cholesterol, and reduced their LDL (bad) cholesterol… and triglycerides (fat in the blood)… between 6 months and 2 years…

The participants admitted to having felt similar levels of fulfilment, satiety, and satisfaction with all diets…

#benefit, #cost, #diet, #disorder, #doctor, #eat, #food, #guide, #heal, #health, #junk, #nutrition, #recipe, #sport, #walk, #weight,

Jesse CRAIGNOU

A reasonable range of fat, proteins and carbons…

The plans didn't include a low in carbon diet type such as Dr Atkins', says Sacks, because people don't keep to low carbon diets and we wanted to remain realistic"…

Research suggests the participants may feel satiated for longer periods while on diets richer in proteins, but those dieters didn't say any difference in their feeling of satiety, says Catherine Loria, a nutritional epidemiologist working for the Lung, Heart and Blood Institute…

Keith Ayoob, a dietician member of Albert Einstein College of Medicine in New York, says that a healthy weight loss is the result of a diet 'over the long run'…

#benefit, #cost, #diet, #disorder, #doctor, #eat, #food, #guide, #heal, #health, #junk, #nutrition, #recipe, #sport, #walk, #weight,

page 28 of 87

Hungry for Diets
Everything you've always wanted to know about diets… and yet were never told !

Jesse CRAIGNOU

AFSSA *study of 15 diets…*

15 diets estimated to be dangerous by the ANSES

See (French) http://www.weightlossforall.com/fr/15-regimes-juges-dangereux-par-lanses.

The French National Agency for Health and Food Security, of the Environment and Work (Anses) –ex AFSSA- published a study assessing the risks linked to dieting back in November 2010. This study rests on scientific expertise, the INCA 2 study, realised in 2006-07 on a sample of the population living in France (1,455 3-17 year old children and 2,624 18-79 year old adults).

The study is generally concerned with diets, the lost popular of which, such as the Dr Dukan's, Dr Cohen's and Montignac's diets, exposing them as bad for health, as they generate lacks and imbalances… which I personally have found to be the exact opposite of what AFSSA claims in the case of Montignac's which promotes variety and balance…

In 65 % of cases, the diet will be followed by a weight gain often in excess of the weight lost during the diet.

The 15 diets studied and questioned are as follows :

- *Dr Atkins's*
- *Californian*
- *Lemon*
- *Dr Delabos Chrononutrition*
- *Dr Cohen's*
- *Dr Dukan's*
- *Dr Fricker's*
- *Mayo*
- *Dr Agatston's Miami*
- *Montignac's*
- *Dr Ornish's*
- *Dr Tarnower's Scarsdale*
- *Cabbage Soup*
- *Weight Watchers*
- *M. Sears's Zone*

We already know a few of them… and their results…

#benefit, #cost, #diet, #disorder, #doctor, #eat, #food, #guide, #heal, #health, #junk, #nutrition, #recipe, #sport, #walk, #weight,

Jesse CRAIGNOU

We suggest you read the conclusions of the report aiming at dieters :

- *The search for weight loss without formal medical prescription bears risks… in particular when the dieter calls upon dietary unbalanced and presenting little or no variety practices. Thus dieting requires a medical prescription and follow-up…*

- *The latter follow-up needs to be adapted to the dieter's status (weight, size, etc.)…*

- *In the absence of weight loss : the diets –whether prescribed by the medical field or not- are risky at best… people should thus be warned of the noxious consequences over the short, mid and long term… as those diets are unbalanced and associated with severe eating disorders… and may lead to a potential irreversible weight gain. The prescription for obesity, weight loss or important weight gain requires a full diagnosis taking into consideration causes, context, and an assessment of the consequences, it requires implementing indication for weight loss and the definition of objectives and means to implement that are not merely restricted to the diet itself… it should aim at an adapted and careful reduction in weight precociously planned (so as to act on the original factors) and then the implementation of a stabilisation plan with the relevant means, while watching the state of physical and psychological health in the mid to long run…*

- *The evolution of dietary habits must be associated to the introduction, the maintenance, or even the augmentation of a regular exercise.*

- *Obesity is a multifactor chronic disease and its cure requires interdisciplinary steps (nutritional medicine, endocrinology, dietician, psychological, etc.)…*

What to do then ?

We have tried to put forward on Weightlossforall, the good point to moderate diets including essential elements for a balanced diet such as in the Paleo, Cretan as well diets with good eating habits to follow like the basic acid and the chewing diet…

The objective of those diets is to protect from civilisation diseases (cancer, chronic fatigue, obesity, etc.). The consequence of a balanced diet and regular exercise will give you better results if you're looking to lose weight, and don't suffer from an

#benefit, #cost, #diet, #disorder, #doctor, #eat, #food, #guide, #heal, #health, #junk, #nutrition, #recipe, #sport, #walk, #weight,

Jesse CRAIGNOU

obesity condition…

If you're suffering from obesity, the recommendations of the study are identical to our recommendation to go and check with a health professional (doctor, dietician, psychologist, endocrinologist, etc.) so as to help and assist you in your progress. You may read our article on obesity if you're suffering from it.

The full study is available on the <u>AFSSA</u> site.

Let me add here that the ANSES shows there is in fact no solution…
It is totally wrong to say that the Montignac diet is unbalanced… as, contrarily to that, it offers to balance our diet back… but of course, Montignac is not a medical professional nor a doctor… and thus will never be done right nor be given street credibility by the health authorities… who have never had the first clue of a solution to offer on their side…

The Montignac diet is one of the only –if not the only- to work effortlessly over the long term… and offers the advantage of being appropriate to any culture or eating habits… as it doesn't withdraw any ingredient (except industrial sugar)… but 'remixes' the ingredients so as to dissociate then for a better metabolisation… and a natural weight loss… in harmony with our body… and lifestyle…

#benefit, #cost, #diet, #disorder, #doctor, #eat, #food, #guide, #heal, #health, #junk, #nutrition, #recipe, #sport, #walk, #weight,

page 31 of 87

Jesse CRAIGNOU

All diets impose a very hard and restrictive discipline for a lifetime… and even while following them we may put weight (back) on… not to mention all those who never lost any weight at all…
We are still waiting for the diet that works over the long run…

Most diets are merely freakish, and tested over the long term, only sport their inefficiency in making dieters lose weight…

The one and only good point to all those diets is to remind us to watch our food and avoid excesses even in dieting excesses…
But above all **reducing and depriving diets don't work because it is not in human nature to deprive people of food or undereat**… but to experiment and do everything possible for survival… as soon as man needs something he goes looking for it… and eventually finds it… and so it goes for the body and metabolism… or for lack of a better idea it finds a substitute… and man has learnt to integrate this as part of his genetics… what's more man is inquisitive AND greedy ! A hunter gatherer by nature…
Eventually every ingredient or food that was ever withdrawn from staple diet in the event of dieting… has been rehabilitated… except for sugar… as (added) sugar is not natural and thus not properly assimilated by the metabolism and body… and that sugar is often replaced by glucose, which is sugar anyway… and 100 years ago nobody ate added sugar… or fat…
Worse still… all those ingredients scorned decades ago have now been found to offer unsuspected benefits… all for the better food and diet… no hats off to the specialists, doctors, dieticians, and nutritionists !
This is but the sad realisation of a total 'scientific' flop… maybe the worst ever… if we don't die of overweight we might at least all die of laughter !

All the partial diets (hips, belly, waist, thighs, men, women, summer, winter, 20+, 50+, after pregnancy, smokers, … the list runs for as long as you like…) take the abovementioned elements with more or less whims and restrictions and… the same results at the bottom line.

Let's just remember the poor imagination our diet suppliers have exhibited and how they have all copied on one another and all claimed a dietary revolution in turn and death to fat… and yet each and every one of them scores a hit every time… some of them are even overweight !
When will we ever learn ? What will it take ?

#benefit, #cost, #diet, #disorder, #doctor, #eat, #food, #guide, #heal, #health, #junk, #nutrition, #recipe, #sport, #walk, #weight,

Hungry for Diets
Everything you've always wanted to know about diets… and yet were never told !

Today the trend goes for a varied diet without any total restriction of any ingredient… the introduction… rather than the exclusion…
Eat 5 fruit and 5 veg everyday… a lost battle for a challenge… as it require enormous logistics and most of us are in fact very loyal to a very narrow range of food… with little variety…

My conclusion has been to compile all in one those miracle diet recipes without noticing the slightest hint of a change…
I have been a vegetarian for more than half of my life (30 years)… without ever noticing any difference or consequence on my body…

And still to date all of those who claim to advise me on my diet have never listened to my story or history… of all of us who is the specialist… when it comes to my body and metabolism ? Who should talk about diet ?
I have collected more experience over the long run than any of them… whichever doctor I might have spoken to… I might even top them all !

Despite their forceful and no nonsense approach, none of their diets has ever brought the definite solution I was looking for in the long run…

#benefit, #cost, #diet, #disorder, #doctor, #eat, #food, #guide, #heal, #health, #junk, #nutrition, #recipe, #sport, #walk, #weight,

page 33 of 87

Jesse CRAIGNOU

Convenience Foods

In a nutshell forget precooked, packed and convenience foods...
They present only disadvantages... and not one advantage...
Too expensive, too small, totally unbalanced, too salty, too sweet, tasteless and lacking ingredients... they often contain a host of chemicals and don't bring the food the dieter's body deserves to feel full and rewarded by a proper meal... Yuck !

And recent events on food fraud point at them too... the contents of their packages is often more than dubious... and you may be facing some unsavoury element when opening the box... putting you off food altogether !

It is easy, simple, and quick to prepare a proper dish... even for the less ready and talented of cooks... and may be as much as 6 times cheaper !

#benefit, #cost, #diet, #disorder, #doctor, #eat, #food, #guide, #heal, #health, #junk, #nutrition, #recipe, #sport, #walk, #weight,

Jesse CRAIGNOU

Miracle Foods

After miracle diets miracle foods…
They just seem to spring up from everywhere all at once… everyone has his own… if not more…

Pineapple
Artichoke
Coffee
Lemon
Water
Hoodia
Maca
Apple
Green tea
To name but a few… in any case, there's always a new one… none of which ever work…
Pineapple burns fat, improves digestion and the digestive track while helping with back problems…

Besides from the fact that the dieter would need to eat tons of it to get a result… the overeating of some food may lead to disaster… starting with a major imbalance in diet… if the dieter can beat the monotony…
Coffee and tea are not good for the nervous system and the heart… lemon can take your teeth away… water may damage your kidneys and liver beyond therapy… the list is never-ending…

As soon as we put the body to test it answers… and usually by burning calories… with the same effect as diets… for a while… and often make dieters and non-dieters happy… boredom is not far… and kilos soon come back… results are only short-lived…
The human body always manages to keep fat stocks one way or another… it's a natural process… and if that fat goes fast and first at the slightest change in eating habits or diet… it is precisely the argument that all the medical field and nutritionists rest their case on… without any form of appeal…

Nobody has ever been able to explain why some of us will eat anything in any quantity and never ever see their weight budge either way… just as some others will undereat or grossly overeat…
My brother has been on a one meal a day staple diet for over 15 years…. and weighs the same as me… he's overweight too… in excess of 40 kilos…

#benefit, #cost, #diet, #disorder, #doctor, #eat, #food, #guide, #heal, #health, #junk, #nutrition, #recipe, #sport, #walk, #weight,

Hungry for Diets

Everything you've always wanted to know about diets… and yet were never told !

Jesse CRAIGNOU

Miracle foods just like miracle diets don't exist…

And if one existed or was ever discovered… everybody would know it… and I'd be the first to get it… the fortune of the discoverer would be assured !

#benefit, #cost, #diet, #disorder, #doctor, #eat, #food, #guide, #heal, #health, #junk, #nutrition, #recipe, #sport, #walk, #weight,

page 36 of 87

Jesse CRAIGNOU

Fasting

Selina weighs 140 kilos… and yet over the past year and a half she's been going to the swimming pool everyday to do her daily 100 lengths… and yet she's still waiting and hoping to shed her first kilo…

She has just discovered fasting and is now fasting 2 days a week… to see her weight drop several kilos every week… regaining control of both her shape and fitness… and will eventually lose 40 kilos… she has never felt so good nor had so much stamina… still she will go on after that as she's hoping to shed another 30 before the summer…

Scorned by many, acclaimed by others, fasting –while at both extremes of reasonable eating and dieting- is gaining momentum again with the results we know… kilos melt away like ice in the sun… and come back as soon as the fast is over…

Fasting comes in many forms… from a total fast 1 day a week over a limited period to a regular 1 to 2 days a week… or 1 meal a day… or avoiding solid food to favour liquids… fasting a week a month for 1 quarter of 1 year… the idea still rests on deprivation and food restriction… that is found in every diet whatever… only this time highly concentrated… remember to make sure you're not overtaken by your fast…

To those who hold out –and why not- reasonable fasting enables regaining lost sensations and the limits of one's body and metabolism… still all those who fast outside a complete ascetism will sooner or later drop it… and go back to their primary condition…

Fasting may be drastic and go along with a health or religious or spiritual discipline… the effects are always the same… that is the faster will maintain his/her fast…

Detoxifiers and drains belong on the same shelf… they offer no durable result and more undesirable side effects than desired… and by the way, it seems that when it comes to eliminate men and women are totally unequal… if men usually go to the stool once or twice a day… women can avoid the stool for a whole week without realising an impact either way on their body, health or weight… even while taking dietary supplements to help eliminate…

Remaining on the chapter of elimination and metabolisation, our stools do not seem to tally without our food intake… even with the same food on the same person…

I was 21 when I was diagnosed with a slow metabolism… my doctor then had warned me that I was to practise sports regularly all my life… or else… sports, is the only really to accelerate the metabolism… on the other hand if sports really do have a positive impact on weight –although many doctors will still tell you otherwise- they

#benefit, #cost, #diet, #disorder, #doctor, #eat, #food, #guide, #heal, #health, #junk, #nutrition, #recipe, #sport, #walk, #weight,

also require a regular practice as well as an increasing practice… or else again the exercising body may still put on weight while keeping the regular exercise up…

#benefit, #cost, #diet, #disorder, #doctor, #eat, #food, #guide, #heal, #health, #junk, #nutrition, #recipe, #sport, #walk, #weight,

page 38 of 87

Jesse CRAIGNOU

Exercise and Sport

There are 2 schools of thought here…
Some are unconditional sports freaks and will go for sports every time while others will tell you sports don't promote weight loss…
And each one will contradict the other… ad libitum… all to no avail…

Exercise is always beneficial and that for many reasons… keeping fit, socialising and discovery…
A sportsman's diet combined with exercise and sports have the same shortcomings as diets… they are not natural to man and are often tedious to practise and soon put off…
Just like Selina, Beverley starves herself for months on end… and has been going swimming for years to do her 100 lengths 2 or 3 times a week and sometimes at weekends… only to get back home with her uncompromising weight…
And just like Beverley, Celine goes jogging and runs every race and marathon she can put her legs to… only to get back home overladen with her excess weight…
Rachelle has long lived off her passion, dancing, which took her all over the world… but two maternities got the better of her good figure, which she hardly ever dares exhibit in public now with the excess 30 kilos she drags around all the time… desperately clinging to her diet and exercise not matter what she does to shed them…
Just like Rachelle, Lina has been exercising daily for 30 years in front of her television screen to the rhythm and the rhyme of Jane Fonda's videos… a lost battle she is now retreating from… giving up as weight hasn't given in yet…

My mother has practised sports all her youth… way beyond 30… overtaxing herself with exercises every morning before a day's work that proves to be very dynamic and very demanding… and kept her excess weight on all the way…

#benefit, #cost, #diet, #disorder, #doctor, #eat, #food, #guide, #heal, #health, #junk, #nutrition, #recipe, #sport, #walk, #weight,

page 39 of 87

Jesse CRAIGNOU

Pills, Powders and other Magic Formulae...

To top up diets there are all the side products claiming to help the dieter lose yet more weight all the faster and the more easily… not only shed weight but eliminate, detoxify, slim, reshape, sculpt, …

They offer a mixed match of magic potions, pills, herbal teas, additives, and other creams and stuff…

The miracle remedies, plants, fruit, which all claim to control, lower, eliminate water and fat… new ones come out by the score every day… in actual facts, results remain impossible to prove or demonstrate… when they're not altogether absent… hope soon takes off and sales drop as fast as they rose…

In the best cases, the dieter would need to take astronomical quantities only to see a minimal effect… and even there undesirable –if not noxious- side effects may be lurking…

Drinking green tea will make you slim and lose weight… if you can drink 80 litres a day ! And I don't need to remind you of the drastic effects of taking too much liquid on the liver and kidneys…

As to me I had tried them by the score without ever noticing the slightest change… the smallest difference… except in my bank account !
No escape there either…
Some of them such as Allì are even dangerous… with more than off-putting undesirable side effects… to say the least…

The pharmaceutical, chemical, cosmetics, and food industries have had us swallow all sorts of a helter skelter mix of odds and ends… with the sole aim of having us consume… under the pretence of taking care of our health and beauty…

All products, which are eventually exposed as health hazards… and are withdrawn from the shelves… sometimes even under much advertised storms and controversies… by the same medias which promoted them !

Medicine and cosmetics come together and exchange roles for the benefits of some laboratories and producers… thus cosmetics are only supposed to remain ON the skin, although most cosmetic creams claim to be easily absorbed by the skin ! If it is absorbed by the skin and or the body in any way it is then classified as medicine… and no longer cosmetics, which an illegal use of the 'medicine' term ! In which case, as a chemical belonging in the medical field… and so it should be approved by state health authorities…

I am always shocked to see the products women (mostly) spread on their body or even swallow… products containing the most lethal of ingredients (lead, mercury, and many other unsavoury chemical mixes)…

#benefit, #cost, #diet, #disorder, #doctor, #eat, #food, #guide, #heal, #health, #junk, #nutrition, #recipe, #sport, #walk, #weight,

Jesse CRAIGNOU

I would just say eat healthy organic fresh products as much as you can… including cereals in your diet… even if real genuine organic food cannot be found on a polluted planet…

#benefit, #cost, #diet, #disorder, #doctor, #eat, #food, #guide, #heal, #health, #junk, #nutrition, #recipe, #sport, #walk, #weight,

page 41 of 87

Jesse CRAIGNOU

Hoodia, L-Carnitine and other Fat Burners

They only make you hungry…
Not only that but their effects remain challenged…
The only benefit of the Hoodia is generating an extra income to the Namibian pygmies…

I have indeed tried them all one after the other… and the only thing that got thinner was my wallet…
To top it all they make your skin dry, hair and nails brittle, and scarring longer and more difficult… they also give permanent pangs of hunger painstakingly and painfully scavenging your inners for the smallest fat…
I have also experienced **severe headaches** while on them… now the brain is made of fat… do these products attack your brain fat ?
It has helped me understand why the Chinese and Asians who eat a lot of Konjac eat all day !

#benefit, #cost, #diet, #disorder, #doctor, #eat, #food, #guide, #heal, #health, #junk, #nutrition, #recipe, #sport, #walk, #weight,

page 42 of 87

Hungry for Diets
Everything you've always wanted to know about diets… and yet were never told !

Jesse CRAIGNOU

Medicine and Alicaments

Medicine is promoted to make us believe they will solve any health problem… including the elimination of our rebel fat… in fact, on top of generating side effects, they do not bring any solution to our overweight issue and that's a massive problem !

#benefit, #cost, #diet, #disorder, #doctor, #eat, #food, #guide, #heal, #health, #junk, #nutrition, #recipe, #sport, #walk, #weight,

page 43 of 87

Jesse CRAIGNOU

Essential Oils

Relaxing, disinfecting, detoxifying, scarring, etc. some are even… but slimming, weight reducing… well… remains to be seen…
Essential oils may relax a person who uses other means to reduce this/her weight… but when it comes to actually doing the reducing… no such luck !

#benefit, #cost, #diet, #disorder, #doctor, #eat, #food, #guide, #heal, #health, #junk, #nutrition, #recipe, #sport, #walk, #weight,

page 44 of 87

Jesse CRAIGNOU

Massages

Massages may help in reducing weight in that they may release blockages of the lymph circulation, perilymph, etc. which are responsible for blockages of certain bodily functions which may result in water retention, intoxications or collection of fat residues…

To look on the bright side, massages bring the benefits of rediscovering body care with a deep impact while relaxing the recipient of the massage as much as the masseur…

#benefit, #cost, #diet, #disorder, #doctor, #eat, #food, #guide, #heal, #health, #junk, #nutrition, #recipe, #sport, #walk, #weight,

page 45 of 87

Jesse CRAIGNOU

Osteopathic Adjustments

Osteopathic adjustments should ideally be a regular practice for all… because we all at one time or another make a wrong move and injure or hurt a part of our body which will need adjusting… and the befits go way beyond weight loss and slimming for reasons close to those described in massages…
Whatever they may be the benefits of osteopathy on the body have long been proved by now… they are general and undeniable…

#benefit, #cost, #diet, #disorder, #doctor, #eat, #food, #guide, #heal, #health, #junk, #nutrition, #recipe, #sport, #walk, #weight,

page 46 of 87

Jesse CRAIGNOU

Slimming Creams

Slimming creams would the miracle remedy for women conscious of their looks… and more and more men are joining them…

If only we weren't presented with model verging on anorexia nervosa to promote them… and then only announcing a reduction measure only in decimals… if supported by a diet… the real message here is : *'Forget slimming creams as they will not give you any results !'* Why bother buying them ?

Their only benefit is the massage you get when applying them…

#benefit, #cost, #diet, #disorder, #doctor, #eat, #food, #guide, #heal, #health, #junk, #nutrition, #recipe, #sport, #walk, #weight,

Jesse CRAIGNOU

Thalassotherapy and Spas

Thalassotherapy surely brings results… but which remain a far cry from expectations and promises… yet the benefits may be like those of massages, shiatsu, … even if the individual indications are different or even remote from the original idea…

#benefit, #cost, #diet, #disorder, #doctor, #eat, #food, #guide, #heal, #health, #junk, #nutrition, #recipe, #sport, #walk, #weight,

page 48 of 87

Jesse CRAIGNOU

Apostles of Sport Ascetics

Sport keeps people fit when practiced reasonably… and enables controlling and maintaining weight through helping to eliminate excess water, fat and sugar…
Yet for those people natural pushed to excess weight and measures the outcome is only kept at bay…

Let's remember that regular sport practice is best when monitor by a professional or a doctor…

#benefit, #cost, #diet, #disorder, #doctor, #eat, #food, #guide, #heal, #health, #junk, #nutrition, #recipe, #sport, #walk, #weight,

page 49 of 87

Jesse CRAIGNOU

Psychological Analysis

The reasons for obesity are not always metabolical… but diabolical…
They may also be found in an event, which may have occurred in the dieter's life… and when the source has been found it can be solved and the dieter will natural return to his/her natural figure…

#benefit, #cost, #diet, #disorder, #doctor, #eat, #food, #guide, #heal, #health, #junk, #nutrition, #recipe, #sport, #walk, #weight,

page 50 of 87

Jesse CRAIGNOU

Medicine

My parents spent their lives on medication and diets !
With every meal the table exhibited a whole chemistry… invading the table more and more as time went by… and with the list of undesirable side effects was getting longer…

One day came my first meeting with my cardiologist… who seals our meeting with writing a long prescription… I ask him how long I was to take all those medicine… and he answers as though to a stupid question… '*For the rest of your life !*'
To which I answer that he's is not curing me… but enlisting me for a lifelong addiction… without the faintest hope of remission… or ever healing… the cure is thus worse than the ailment… silence… the all-knowing doctor hasn't got it in him to answer a pertinent question…
I am talking of a child who has never seen his parents not take medicine !
How is that child supposed to believe in the benefits of medication ? And/or not be worried about addiction ?

Medicine doesn't bring the answer either ! Allì and Acomplia first acclaimed for their performance were soon to be exposed for their lack of proper results… and their most undesirable side effects…
'*And to think those are preventive medicine… for people who are not ill and yet may be*… (Dr Even blows his whistle) *and yet again may never be cured !*'

#benefit, #cost, #diet, #disorder, #doctor, #eat, #food, #guide, #heal, #health, #junk, #nutrition, #recipe, #sport, #walk, #weight,

page 51 of 87

Jesse CRAIGNOU

Plastic Surgery

Plastic surgery, rather expensive if not included in a national health plan, offers a radical and often permanent solution to overweight… when included in a health plan, the patient may have to wait up to 2 years… to get his/her operation… which is submitted to a strict follow-up… some patients might lose their patience when they have already been waiting most –if not all- their life… and the cost may be left to them…

Plastic surgery offers such solutions as the gastric band, the gastric bypass, and the sleeve… the gastric band enables a scheduled tightening of the stomach, the gastric bypass bypasses the stomach to link the oesophagus directly to the small intestine avoiding the stomach altogether, and the sleeve offers a substitution of the stomach… which is probably the most drastic or desperate approach… to my mind at least…

My sister ended up go for an operation and the magic of a bypass… so tired she was of wasting her time and efforts… melting 2 thirds of her body mass away in a couple of months… …

Carol, after 2 years of a medical, nutritional and psychological follow-up… was eventually granted an operation which had been opted for the gastric band… all she can eat for every meal now would fill a teacup… provided she doesn't drink with her meal… as soon as she has lost enough weight she will be eligible for cosmetic surgery… except for the breasts… which will be her to pay for… as this operation is considered purely cosmetic and not medical… after a few operations she's hoping to get her life back…
The drawback with this kind of surgery is it causes damages elsewhere in the body… doctors are now talking about 'deep fat'… which is fat going to the deepest recesses of the muscles… and virtually impossible to get to… looking and digging further…

The one and only last forlorn hope when you've tried everything…
I would go as far as saying that the patient needs to be absolutely sure this is the one and best solution to be granted to the patient…
Plastic surgery often offers the advantage of looking for the 'mechanical' causes of the trouble at hand… and to 'repair' the damage in its own way… with a long term solution if not permanent… without the inconvenience of a chemical addiction or alienation… although it also comes with its side effects… as we know today the unsavoury psychological consequences… even if most of them escape those…

Without listing here all the inconveniences and dangers of exaggerated sports practice… whether under supervision or not, sports people often resort to taking all sorts of stuff, food, tablets and pills, dietary supplement and drugs of all kinds… and the mere fact that sports people reach overweight in their forties up… is another proof that sports or not comes a time of reckoning with the body and metabolism… when the gene deal is non renegotiable…

#benefit, #cost, #diet, #disorder, #doctor, #eat, #food, #guide, #heal, #health, #junk, #nutrition, #recipe, #sport, #walk, #weight,

Jesse CRAIGNOU

Most reasonable diets promote reasonable eating habits and a nutritional rehab... which may be desirable... when accompanied by a (re)discovery of food and the pleasure to eat various types of foods...

To finish, the promises claimed by dietary supplements and other miracles recipes such as the Moon Diet, the Cold Diet, the Stars Diet, the Model Diet, the Cabbage Soup Diet, the Brown Rice Diet, the With Diets, and the Without Diets do not deliver any result worth mention or promoting here... whether in the short, mid, or long term...

As to dietary supplements, hunger cheaters, fat burners, vitamins, and all other detoxifiers and supplements, the body will react in its own unpredictable way... eliminating everything it doesn't recognize, wants or needs (as per its own make-up)... nothing bringing any solution...

And remember most of them would require being taken in astronomical quantities... still without the faintest guarantee of ever bearing fruit... whether in weight loss, weight control or health... even if natural or organic as opposed to chemical...

It seems more and more effects–when they appear at all, whatever small they may be- disappear with age...

More and more studies –and in more and more countries- are made in the hope of proving the validity of supplementation to prove that most of them are in fact totally useless...

I have been reading all those I could cast my eyes on in many languages over the past 30 years...

Any quantification amounts to inviting a bigger consumption... and starving people only makes people eat !

Dr Salman, a French doctor and dietician on a French radio station repeated : 95 % of dieters to their weight back on within weeks of dieting Apr 8 2015... and yet the entire medical field still heavily promotes diets !

This may explain why more and more overweight people, dieters and doctors resort to plastic surgery... which seems to offer the only viable results overall... even if plastic surgery also recommends a healthy lifestyle... sleeves and bypasses impose a substantial reduction in the serving... and ingestion...

My advice would be get extensive information on the practitioner... if only to avoid excesses and abuse...

Whatever the issue and your choice may be push your doctor and nutritionists to their limits... otherwise they'll just put you on any old diet...

#benefit, #cost, #diet, #disorder, #doctor, #eat, #food, #guide, #heal, #health, #junk, #nutrition, #recipe, #sport, #walk, #weight,

Jesse CRAIGNOU

Cellulitis

Cellulitis is natural process that enables stocking for a rainy day… to release in lean periods… which also means that going on a diet you may find that your metabolism retains most of whatever little you eat… and still put on weight… or at least not shed any… nature's way…
Cellulitis may be treated but not done away with altogether…

Some appropriate massages offer a real reduction but never durable… if not kept up all your life…
Still cellulitis may be dealt with effectively through surgery… at least in parts…

#benefit, #cost, #diet, #disorder, #doctor, #eat, #food, #guide, #heal, #health, #junk, #nutrition, #recipe, #sport, #walk, #weight,

page 54 of 87

Jesse CRAIGNOU

Fat Nature Lean Nature – Heavy Kilos Light Kilos

As a child I wanted to become a plastic surgeon… and so I never stopped looking at people of all ages and all types…

All through my observations I have noticed there are various physical types, which are always slim and never put on weight whatever they may eat or do… while others put on weight and never lose it regardless of whatever they may eat or do…

Truth of the pudding is whatever their type and metabolism… there are things that will never change… thus having even having lost 30 kilos, my skeleton remained the same size and I had to make do with what I had…

There are people with slim or small features… and people with big features… tall and lank or short and chunky… the long and lank ones will remain slim while the short and chunky will tend to go the other way… no two ways about it ! And your face will tell the same tale…

Likewise… I have always be regarded as overweight… even while being very slim… my features betrayed me… others -while not so slim- will always be considered slim…

Sex symbol Marylyn Monroe was a size 34 ! Nobody would want her to model today in our days of anorexic models…

As to feeling satiated or not… how many slim people will feel heavy… why other overweight people feel light… doctors and nutritionists and other dieticians take one look at me and scorn me for making a pig of myself stuffing my face any way I can… when I never overeat… in fact I eat less than most people I share my table with… I feel bloated very quickly… and seeing a lot of food makes me feel sick… let alone eat it…

We each and all have our own type and style… and too often do we conform to standards that are not our own… but other people's… or the passing trend, fashion, cosmetics, industry, and the food industry… we're sacrificed to the business at hand… but whatever we do or think deep down we remain ourselves…

Eventually having come of age, I noticed and learnt that there are hair types that indicate this one will lose his hair and that one won't… while some people's hair will curl and others' will remain desperately straight… there are those bodies that will put on weight and others that won't… and will keep making muscles while others only seem to make fat…

And again nothing we have been offered or proffered has been able to change the deal… or turn the tables either way…

We have all seen all the homeless squatting public places everywhere or under a makeshift shelter somewhere… they are all put up in the own way… they all have to put up with the same diet… and still some are bigger than others… from the slimmest to the biggest… no slim person has ever been told off for eating junk or fat food… or anything unbalanced… and yet there are indeed a lot of slim people out there who constantly eat the food fat people wouldn't been seen dead with !

#benefit, #cost, #diet, #disorder, #doctor, #eat, #food, #guide, #heal, #health, #junk, #nutrition, #recipe, #sport, #walk, #weight,

Hungry for Diets
Everything you've always wanted to know about diets… and yet were never told !

Jesse CRAIGNOU

We are never told that most of the cholesterol we have in our body is the one we produce… and has nothing to do with what we eat…

We are constantly told that our excess cholesterol is the result of our lack of exercise, of food too rich in fat, sugar and alcohol… whereas traces of atherosclerosis and cholesterol have been found in the bodies of Egyptian mummies… which goes to prove that theory wrong ! Ancient Egyptians cannot be blamed for their lack of exercise and eating too rich food…

A diet is usually a waste of time there again…

My niece in Hong Kong was a stunning beauty !

She had the small size many Asian have… while her parents are tall and big… and her elder brother is grossly overweight… the moment she turned 8 she blew up like a balloon… to go on and look the same as the rest of her family… without any hope of return…

In 2014 a study carried by Stanford University revealed that the daily food intake of the average American hadn't changed since the sixties… and that if they were overweight today… it was due to a lack of exercise… and yet…

Aged 25 Andrew is the size of 3 adults… yet he has been a great sports teacher for years in his sports club in a small town in the North of England…

Martina, 32, is a hyperactive midget and the life and soul of the party…

One day while I take her food to her table she tells me she on a very strict fat free diet… *'Yes… she sighs… I weigh 37.5 kilos and I'm on a strict diet… unbelievable but true'…*

Alice, 35, has practiced running for years, compiling breath-taking training sessions and competitions… sporting just like her twin sister, who has never practised any sports, an overweight figure out of control despite the repeated diets she's been on for half her life…

Anne, 37, has tried every diet under the sun… yet her body persists in coming back to her overweight… no matter how hard she tries…

She has never overeaten and her staple diet is balanced… it was her who introduced me to Montignac… and we had both melted… once upon a time…

Celine is almost 40… she stopped smoking 2 years ago… and to fight the pangs started running every day… running marathons several times a year and all the preparation and practice in between… yet she has never been able to shed all those extra kilos that make choosing and buying the clothes she loves an ordeal…

If physical exercise is a good thing for some… one practice doesn't fit all… and we all know that sports professional put on weight when they retire… as their overtaxed body, used to overproduce to meet the calorie cost of their efforts, hasn't stopped production when they stopped practising…

#benefit, #cost, #diet, #disorder, #doctor, #eat, #food, #guide, #heal, #health, #junk, #nutrition, #recipe, #sport, #walk, #weight,

Jesse CRAIGNOU

My cousin Nathalie is tiptoeing to her 50th birthday… dragging along a 30 kilo excess luggage… she has been towing for the past 25 years… having suffered an intense emotional stress as a young mother she used to make herself throw up all the food she took for 10 years without ever shedding a gram !

Patrick, 55 has kept his teenage body all the way up and down his 6.5 foot height and still wears the 2 pairs of jeans he bought when he was 16… still his cholesterol level is under high watch as it keeps overflowing… although he tends to eat more than reasonably… and has been on a balanced diet all life…

A teacher at the world famous school of the Paris Opera repeated in an interview : '*We recruit on the bases of long and slim body lines… as they are those which tend to remain slim*'… Ditto ! Like I noticed decades before as a teenager…

To date no doctor, no scientist has ever researched into how and why the body manages its resources and its weight… and no GP ever asks us about our linage or family history… before turning our food against us…
Progress would mean face those accusations and blames patients are charged with…

We are shown monsters exhibited in a freak show… people eating masses of metal… that their body metabolises happily… without any consequence whatsoever on their health and body… if not for the better…
How much more time will it take for nature to take a keen interest in them ?

Yet science knows so many things… things it tells us again and again… over and over again and again…
Astronomers tell us that weight may vary depending on gravity and intensity… and if so on earth why not men ?

#benefit, #cost, #diet, #disorder, #doctor, #eat, #food, #guide, #heal, #health, #junk, #nutrition, #recipe, #sport, #walk, #weight,

page 57 of 87

Jesse CRAIGNOU

Cholesterol

Research and progress show us more and more how man tends to collect more and more cholesterol… in a major statistical way that spreads over all the layers of society and mankind… way up from the dawn of mankind to modern man…

But cholesterol is produced by the body and not –or only so little- collected from our food intake which our body generally disposes of… and yet nobody has looked into the causes… rather than the consequences… and systematically summon the patient to a strict diet… with the poor results we know… a diet that will never yield the promised results… as the cholesterol that weighs us down does not come from our food !

Last but not least, cholesterol is a metabolical production… which comes to compensate for the loss of plasticity of our aging and breaking veins… even if our production soars undesirably at times…

This goes to prove why no doctor has ever been able to prescribe a working treatment… you might as well try and stop the wind…

Doctors are happy repeated old doctors' tales… doctors don't seem to agree on diets or food steps to take… they have remained unable to offer a personal diet… as I was saying earlier no doctor today ask his/her patient about the family history as was done in the past… and if you bully them into giving you a relevant piece of information they have nothing decent to offer…

#benefit, #cost, #diet, #disorder, #doctor, #eat, #food, #guide, #heal, #health, #junk, #nutrition, #recipe, #sport, #walk, #weight,

page 58 of 87

Jesse CRAIGNOU

Quantity

When I was 25 I used to order a big salad, a pizza and a dessert with half bottle of wine… half a bottle of mineral water and a coffee… and back then my weight didn't budge…
Today when I've had a pizza and a mineral water I feel like a crocodile who's just had an elephant for lunch…

In the 50s and 60s Diana DORS, the British answer to Marilyn Monroe, is at the top of her career envied or copied by women and desired by men… for her beauty…
A bubbly blonde, she flaunt her then wasp waist… without ever letting on she starves herself all the time… till the day she decided she had had more than enough and was going to live her life… and let her body take over the space around her to the point of losing herself in her own weight… a far cry from the beauty standards she had contributed to impose…
She will eventually die at a relatively young age, very ill, and unhappy… may she rest in peace…

Bubbly and shapely Anita Ekberg has had generations of men dream about her… her scene in La Dolce Vita will have her remembered forever and enter the realm of the cinema pantheon… with her unforgettable 'Marcello'… Most people won't ever know the once Miss Sweden spent most of her life warding kilos and fighting for her weight… kilos and weight that never really let go off her…

Like them, Nelly, Catherine, Olivier, Yochanon, Patrick and so many others fought till their last breath… only to get to the same result… none !

All the diets, which promoted reducing the size of portions have long given up on the idea…

Hungry for Diets
Everything you've always wanted to know about diets… and yet were never told !

Jesse CRAIGNOU

I eventually change GP again… and my new doctor takes stock on my situation… asking me about my parents and my family… for the first time in my patient's life… the first and only doctor in over a dozen… to ever ask me…

She confirms what I had told each and everyone of them : all the people who suffer from heart problems put on weight (almost 2 years before I almost died and went into a coma from a massive lung oedema !)… whereas all the others had told me otherwise… that it wasn't true… that men didn't suffer from water retention… and that the only reason I was overweight is I was overeating and probably unbalanced and junk food !

#benefit, #cost, #diet, #disorder, #doctor, #eat, #food, #guide, #heal, #health, #junk, #nutrition, #recipe, #sport, #walk, #weight,

page 60 of 87

Jesse CRAIGNOU

Food and Evolution

It is clear that today our food is also the fruit of our evolution… and the same goes for the way our body metabolises our food intake… takes or leaves our eating…
We are often told what we should not eat… but never told what we should eat…

Thus the Neanderthal man would have had more gut than the modern man… until he cooked his meat… which seems to apply to my vegetarian diet which blew up all the time with gas… until I took some meat 20 years later (since then dropped again)…
Let's all remember that carbon in small doses is good for the digestive track…

Nature always wins…
We all tend to be fatter in winter than in summer…
After a liposuction fat comes back in another place often in equal measures…

The preconceived ideas of :
- Food & health, fitness
- Intense physical exercise
- Beauty and well-being status and definitions

Are begging to be revised or revisited… if not altogether abolished…

I have seen people diet all their lives…
Couldn't we just agree to the fact that there are men and women who have other sizes ? Just as there are men and women who have other sizes… other sprouts of humanity which have disappear… or have been wiped off the face of the planet… men and women of other types or other colours…
Shouldn't we just revisit our health and shape criteria ?

Besides, we also know that mithridatisation enables insects to evolve quickly by developing new talents and skills… and newly found resistance to treatment or insecticides… ants and termites excel at the art of forming a whole colony segmented into extremely varied individuals to meet the requirement of the whole community… and all the different breeds of dogs come from one wolf !

This is also true of humans !
The difference –at least that noticed in humans- is that evolution comes quickly… but that regression is very slow in comparison to progress… when possible at all… yet doesn't ever seem to happen…
Everything happens as though our evolution was programmed to go one way… with all the collaterals pros and cons it involves as a consequence… thus all the new human 'acquisitions' would not necessarily be in favour of being slim and light… Let's imagine for a moment that our gravity was lowering… and we would need to be heavier in order to be able to make-up for the loss and enjoy living on planet Earth…
Food for thought…

#benefit, #cost, #diet, #disorder, #doctor, #eat, #food, #guide, #heal, #health, #junk, #nutrition, #recipe, #sport, #walk, #weight,

Jesse CRAIGNOU

Thyroid Test

I would recommend before anything to have the thyroid activity tested… the same goes for food intolerances and anything, which may reveal a cause or an origin bringing on a weight gain… although this does seem to be ever done…

First things first… every time I asked to have such tests done I was discouraged… and my suggestion ignored…

#benefit, #cost, #diet, #disorder, #doctor, #eat, #food, #guide, #heal, #health, #junk, #nutrition, #recipe, #sport, #walk, #weight,

page 62 of 87

Jesse CRAIGNOU

Genetics

Not one diet takes into account the genetics of the dieter…
Not one diet is successful over the long run…

All the diets make people lose weight at the beginning… as the mere fact of changing diet make the metabolism adjust and overreact… which causes a hopeful weight loss at the beginning and false hope for the dieter thus led to believe that diet is the solution to his weight management… yet 95 % of dieters regain the weight loss within a maximum of 2 years… and sometimes they put back on much more than they had to begin with… causing all the more despair… and paving the way for the Yoyo effect…
The only dieters for whom a diet works are those who grossly overate and had an unbalanced diet…
No diet will work for everyone… on the head of one individual the hair doesn't grow at the same speed… and each individual hair grows at its own speed… the same goes for humans…

Genetics progresses in leaps and bounds… and faster and faster…
It has shown us that nature is here to stay and nature will always win…

In the 90s we believed that our children were growing taller and taller beyond the average size –strangely a belief that seems limited to France-… people thought they had detected evolution there until it was shown that excessive use and prescription of antibiotics –again very common in France- were the cause for this 'growth'… further along the line of growth it was shown that this growth was not growth… as it didn't apply to all the children but only a few… and that an equal proportion of short children remained as per human evolution and history…
Antibiotics had the nasty tendency to inhibit growth hormone regulation and promote growth hormones, which may lead to other health issues eventually…

#benefit, #cost, #diet, #disorder, #doctor, #eat, #food, #guide, #heal, #health, #junk, #nutrition, #recipe, #sport, #walk, #weight,

page 63 of 87

Jesse CRAIGNOU

Health and Care Costs

Any patient undergoing hospital treatment or surgery is instantly and upon entry submitted to a diet of one sort or another... but when it is obvious the patient is a victim of his/her overweight is the root of his/her troubles weight reduction surgery is never applied... while it would seem obvious that it should be part of the treatment... the patient would be all the better all the sooner... and go back to work in full shape... and contributing to the contribution to health... as opposed to having a patient depending on health service for the rest of his/her life... in lethargy with his/her weight problems...

Such an approach would same ample expenditure to no avail for the Health Authorities... not to mention the saving in useless paper work and administration... a spending forever increasing... just like all the health problems...

But the cost of health and care is way below the benefits of illness !
Those laboratories which produce medicine are much better off keeping us just below the health line so we continue taking their drugs... that's where all the big money is... healing patients would be the ruin and the death of laboratories !

#benefit, #cost, #diet, #disorder, #doctor, #eat, #food, #guide, #heal, #health, #junk, #nutrition, #recipe, #sport, #walk, #weight,

Jesse CRAIGNOU

What Works

All the medical and nutrition specialists will tell you : *'All the diets will work… for a while… all the dieters have gone back to their overweight within 2 years… when they haven't put on more weight than they had to shed to start with'*…
The gain is far from the pain…

In September 2014 The Journal of American Medicine Association published the results attained by 7, 000 people on 48 different diets… over 6 months… the average loss was only 2-3 kilos…
And every time a miracle diet comes out… it is only the proof that 1 diet worked for 1 person… at least for a while… and not a universal panacea…
The book will sell millions of copies… and make the writer's bank account only fatter…

I have seen people from the whole world eat various types of foods and diets, other diets or other people's…and noticed that at the end of the day there is little –if any- difference between them… which can only leave a fat lot of doubts on the relevance of diets…

An American university study tested 811 people divided into 4 groups… dieting on the freedom of sugar, starch, fats, or other ingredients… to show over, 2 years that they had all lost weight in the same proportion…
I have had to resort to using my own body as a metabolical laboratory… and, having tried every ingredient and food or diet under the sun, realised no food or ingredient is better of worse than any other… so long as people don't overeat or binge all the time…

Besides all that, no doctor, nutritionist, or dietician, has even controlled what they preach over the long term… nor even attempted to see what the opposite of diet might bring… as to me, neither one nor the other seems to have the least effect…

The people who have lost a minimum weight with one or another diet have become reformed moralists and preachers… they will swear given half a chance that THEY have THE solution… and that you don't know what you're talking about… or blatantly lie !
Justice is they will soon learn their lesson and have put whatever weight they claim to have lost back on…

Bridget, 25, dreams of that top model look and figure… her younger brother and sister look just the way she would love to… if only… nature hadn't seen to it otherwise… her mother is short and slim but it seems Bridget has inherited her father's much fuller figure…

Federica, 40, has recently put on 30 kilos in under 2 years…

#benefit, #cost, #diet, #disorder, #doctor, #eat, #food, #guide, #heal, #health, #junk, #nutrition, #recipe, #sport, #walk, #weight,

Jesse CRAIGNOU

She has to relocate to Russia… where her husband had been sent to work on a 5-year contract… the good thing for her is she comes back after 2 years looking like those Russian top model…

She tells me she could never adjust to the Russian diet and never liked their food… and dropped the meat as it was bad quality for fish… and melted some 35 kilos away…

For lack of any results to show I decided to add a few fruit and veg known for the slimming qualities to my staple diet… yet besides the pleasure of eating them, not the slightest weight loss in sight…

Bloated ? Not bloated ?
From my origins, travels and tastes I have been led to taste all types of food, all sorts of cooking methods… and if not all certainly most of them…

I noticed the cooking I was served, although using similar ingredients as any other, had my stomach react in a completely different way… without my ever understanding why the response could come so varied from the same ingredients… how versatile my digestive tract could get depending on whichever cuisine I ate…
Some ingredients have been bloated in no time… while others never do…

Russian and Indian foods take me to satiety without any trouble… no matter how much I eat of it I always feel great… should I give up all the other foods ? Surely the ingredients and the way those people prepare their food has something to do with the way I feel…
North African food satiates me but my digestion is easy… Chinese food blows me up like a balloon and makes me feel like I weigh tons over the one meal…
Eating taboulé (Lebanese semolina salad) dehydrates to the point of calling emergency… while I have a severe water retention condition… it appears I am begging to revisit my water management metabolical system…
Who can tell whether there might be something in it… as the Cretan or Japanese diets are supposed to do…

Whatever it may be we process better the food that comes from our culture… our metabolism adapts all along the generation down the line to what we get used to eating… and what we eat less of is more poorly processed by our system… only I'm not Russian nor Indian…

Jeffrey GORDON tells us that gaining or losing weight depends much on what is in our intestines… only I could have told you that !
He recommends we eat less sugar les sugar and more fibre… which is precisely what I've done most of my life… to no avail… sadly he doesn't answer the question he asks… and if diet rich in fibre are not good for all of us… they don't seem to at least help us shed weight either… nor slim us down… far from it…

The best way to stop cravings is usually detoxifying… thyme tea is the diet's best friend… as it detoxifies the body while topping up in useful minerals… thyme tea is

#benefit, #cost, #diet, #disorder, #doctor, #eat, #food, #guide, #heal, #health, #junk, #nutrition, #recipe, #sport, #walk, #weight,

Jesse CRAIGNOU

also great for digestion, to fight acne and unsightly spots, as well as lazy bowel movement… the more detoxified the body is the less it makes you crave for bad things… naturally… and if taken with a little exercise it will mobilises all the bodily functions, all the organs… while helping to promote good health…

It is sure that some foods and diets, while they don't give results in the long run, may exercise an encouraging effect at the beginning and see the diet engage in regular exercise… which will promote fitness and help the dieter lose weight in the process…

Regular exercise is not the key a to a slim body… a lot of people who exercise are far from slim… walking is a healthy exercise yet in an hour's walk the walker will lose the amount of calories he will get drinking a glass of water at the end of his walk…

Yet regular daily walks promote weight loss… whether walking or Scandinavian (fast stepped) walking… provided you walk everyday…

I always recommend dropping cars and public transport as much as can be done… you will save a lot of money and pollute less !

The diet that works is not a diet… it's logics… and logistics…

If you feel you overeat or have an unbalanced diet… and are prone to cravings… start by eliminating all the excesses you can… and you should at least feel all the better for it… not to mention making a substantial saving…

Exercise as much as you can… it will help you eliminate unwanted weight… and keeping you busy also takes your mind off eating, off fighting your cravings, off living altogether to eat… and you will make new friends…

Nobody in the business or elsewhere is able to tell us what to eat or what not to eat…. The debate on food and health and diets is still raging on… and has been raging for over 100 years ! And every 10 years a miracle therapy comes out… only to be debunked over the following decade…

Nutritionists, dieticians and doctors have all come back on their words over time… the potato, evil food to be banned in the 60 s and 70s has been rehabilitated for its nutritional value, light weight and fibre… and is now highly recommended in diets !

All forbidden whatever the condition or the health problem or ailment… whether overweight, heart trouble, nerve problem, osteoporosis, or else… which goes to prove all the more how irrelevant they are…

Forbidden food our elders ate without any restriction and felt all the better for…

We have known for a long time that our body eliminates every excess or anything that doesn't agree with it… it's inbred in its genetics and human nature… so why not weight excesses and cholesterol ?

The more the chemical and medical industries progress the more ingredients and foods are withdrawn from our diet… and the more ingredients are reintroduced in our diet… for the same reasons they have been withdrawn… yet nobody has ever worried about additives or food substitutes we are force fed under various forms and for various reasons… the same goes for cosmetics which contain aberrations that our body absorbs and integrates through our pores…

#benefit, #cost, #diet, #disorder, #doctor, #eat, #food, #guide, #heal, #health, #junk, #nutrition, #recipe, #sport, #walk, #weight,

Hungry for Diets
Everything you've always wanted to know about diets… and yet were never told !

Jesse CRAIGNOU

All the nutrition industry rests on excess and aberration in eating habits… and regulation of food intake… in its own favourable way… yet nobody has ever wondered whether that might be the root of the problem… which they obviously don't seem to be…

Run from prepacked and convenience foods and meals !
They only offer poorly nutritious and tasteless deals, largely substituting food and flavour in favour of starch and sugar loaded with chemicals… sandwiches are also loaded with poor quality butter and margarines… especially French style sandwiches… which are mostly starch, sugar and fat of next to no nutritious value… Worse still… they are usually made with chemicals and are full of pesticides !

All the same… run from all *'light'* and *'sugar free'* ingredients… *'light'* ingredients often contain a substitute which is in fact water (to avoid in the event of water retention)… sugar is replaced by other sugars or sugary materials…

It is easy even for a poor cook to prepare simple savoury dishes at a low cost… dishes, which will promote health and generate savings… in the dieter's wallet as much as on his/her weight !
Let's remember that the less we pay for our food in food shelves the lower the quality… and the less the good ingredients…

The latest food scandals should be enough to remind us what we are exposed to… Mad Cows Disease, salmonella, the Horsemeat Gate, … one after the other to remind us they came from more than dubious sources… and ingredients such as minced bones… they are all reasons that brought on such things as Mad Cows Disease (foretold 100 years before by Rudolph Steiner)… imagine the impact on humans !
American and European food regulations do nothing to help… they only serve their own interests… the more we regiment and withdraw elements of our diets the more nutritional values we take out… promoting health hazards… this brought about the salmonella crisis… which only happened as the food industry had withdraw the salmonella natural enemy… enabling salmonella to propagate in our food… giving way to a epidemic…

The Franco-Brit in me remembers how my French cousins in the 70s found people in Britain often bigger than their French counterparts… France a kept its agriculture traditional until then while the UK had opted for more productive farming… with all the chemicals it entails… Today's France is on a par with Britain…

Always make sure you eat healthy food… or as healthy as you can…
No one knows what those chemicals may do to your body… GMOs can wreck havoc on a healthy eater… and you can bet your bottom dollar that convenience food is the first place to find them in scores…
Sadly eating organic foods brings no guarantee that your food will be healthier… we have reached a stage at which we have polluted the whole planet so much… pollution and chemicals have reached the furthest and deepest reaches of our home… usually driven by wind and water…

#benefit, #cost, #diet, #disorder, #doctor, #eat, #food, #guide, #heal, #health, #junk, #nutrition, #recipe, #sport, #walk, #weight,

Jesse CRAIGNOU

The other thing is there is no real nor proper regulation of 'organic food'… anyone can label their food as organic without ever being controlled… and organic is not described the same in difference places… and countries… and most shops whether organic or not just get their foods from the same suppliers…
And how can one claim to eat organic on a polluted planet ?

Get as much of your food as possible from a supplier you know and you know have he/she produces their goods… or, better still, start your own garden… it's easy and cheap !

One thing is certain… for the past 50 years I have been studying the subject… and the more I progress in my research… and the more people I meet the more obvious it is that nobody has the answer to weight control… sooner or later your body catches up with you… and creeps up on you…
If your excess weight doesn't arise from aberrant eating habits then there's next to no chance you'll loose it… or only to pick it up again… as that weight is written in the stone of your bones…

Man is more inclined to follow his passion that reason… he soon forgets his good resolutions and drop a mean and lean diet that doesn't deliver what it promised…

#benefit, #cost, #diet, #disorder, #doctor, #eat, #food, #guide, #heal, #health, #junk, #nutrition, #recipe, #sport, #walk, #weight,

Jesse CRAIGNOU

And so what of Underweight People ?

We are often put the question for overweight people… fat obese people… but never for underweight, skinny, bony people… as they too have their own weight problems… There are people in this world who, no matter what or how much they eat, will never have their weight budge either way… underweight people are also people who may not be happy with their weight… and exhibit it…

Japanese people undereat as some people ion the aristocracy used to do… or religious Christians also did for a long time… and then there are macrobiotics and their freaks… it hasn't yet been studied whether undereating has an impact or the weight or the general health of the individual… nor on their longevity or comfort and happiness…

It is high time we looked a the psychological aspects of health…

#benefit, #cost, #diet, #disorder, #doctor, #eat, #food, #guide, #heal, #health, #junk, #nutrition, #recipe, #sport, #walk, #weight,

Jesse CRAIGNOU

Anorexia

Worse still than suffering of excess weight is believing you are overweight… when you're not !
We all know this… anorexia kills…
It killed a young top model, who even modelled to advertise the dangers of anorexia… and Karen Carpenter in full bloom… to name but 2… the music world will never be the same without Karen Carpenter… and the world is never the same for anyone who has lost a dear one…

Women are often prey to anorexia… and women often see themselves as overweight when they're not… even the slimmest and the underweight women…
Ladies beware… magazines are not to be trusted when they tell you what you should look like…

#benefit, #cost, #diet, #disorder, #doctor, #eat, #food, #guide, #heal, #health, #junk, #nutrition, #recipe, #sport, #walk, #weight,

Jesse CRAIGNOU

At the End of the Day

All the medics and paramedics may sing in choir that fat, salt, sugar, and excess weight are bad for the heart… but nobody ever tells us that it is in fact heart problems that may cause the overweight ! Or that most people who have heart problems are not over weight… and most people who die of heart problems are not overweight… because there is no definite response no treatment to heart problems… we are not told so they don't have to tell us the truth…

My cardiologist eventually had to admit, after years of seeing me, that I couldn't lose weight –or at least not much- as my weight problem was caused because of my heart problems…

The same people who constantly harass their patients because our cholesterol comes from eating to much sugar and fat… without ever telling us that the cholesterol we have in our body is the one we produce… and that dieting will not reduce that cholesterol… warding off cholesterol is a lifelong losing battle… as the cholesterol we produce rises with age as it comes to protect our blood vessels !

To carry out a proper study on the effects of food on man would require millions of dollars, thousands of candidates and… a whole life !

Man created a fatal combination in mixing sugar and fat… which turns into addiction… and we all know how bad it is and od not need nor like to be remembered… but do most overweight people in the world live on donuts ?

What matters most here is to have a balanced diet and exercise… but yet again most overweight people eating balanced meals…

Most people will go for taking medicine… as that is the easy way out… despite the frightful side effects… including those causing endocrinal disorders… and may be the cause of weight gain !

One of the main reasons for diet and weight loss failure in the long run is… that people don't always feel like always eating this or that… because it is good for their figure and keeps their weight down… but what they feel like eating for eating pleasure and satiety…

Or at least what they enjoy eating…

The only slimming and/or weight control diet that even work -when they do- are those for people who have bad eating habits, who eat in excess, this evidence goes on to make doctors and nutritionists believe that anyone who is overweight eats like a horse ! And thus should reason and lessen his food… while take more exercise… the only trouble with this is… diet are not the answer and won't ever work ! Never !

Not everybody is the same… and no 2 people have the same genetic make-up… even twins… that eventually makes us who we are… and can't be changed… it will always have the last word…

#benefit, #cost, #diet, #disorder, #doctor, #eat, #food, #guide, #heal, #health, #junk, #nutrition, #recipe, #sport, #walk, #weight,

Jesse CRAIGNOU

At best... food and dietary supplements, which are claimed to have wondrous effects, only really have a placebo effect for most of them...

At worst... they have no effect if only to disturb our metabolism all the more... while creating more problems for us... and it would mean anyway swallowing tons of them and all the time... for them to have an effective benefit... which is not of the possibility or the taste of all... and least yet affordable to all...

Let's just remember that everything we put in our body is generally meant to be there in sufficient quantities (nature is the master) and if it is not needed because it is already there in sufficient quantity and so it will not be kept... or else it will generate an imbalance... as it is no meant top be there or in such quantity...

Comparative studies on superaliment diets show that their impact is generally more negative than positive... your metabolism will only keep what it needs in the quantities it needs them... and no more... likewise all synthetic chemicals are rejected by our metabolism... and this explains why we need such big quantities of them for them to work and have a beneficial effect on us...

As to statistics... besides the fact that they can be interpreted in any sort of way... they never take into account the simple fact that we may all react in our own way and so differently from being to being... our genetics rule our metabolism...

When we go from one study to another we realise they all end up contradicting one another...

There are as many statistics as one may count or account for in most countries... which amount to, at best, show they come to contradictory conclusions or, at worse, to no avail...

In any case, studies more often that not rest on a few dozen cases, may hundreds... when they're not only carried out on animals ! When we would really need hundreds and thousands to be really conclusive...

There are over 7 billion people on earth... rules cannot apply to all of us...

Not one week goes by without hearing talks about the dangers of this or that medicine... which are still prescribed to patients... sometimes for decades... if a genuine medicine existed everybody would know it... and overweight would be history now... and the inventor a rich man... or woman !

There is definitely too much to gain there...

Organic claims to make us eat more healthy food... but nobody again has ever proved it... and again the planet is so polluted that it is impossible to grow organic food... even if we try and avoid all pollutants...

In any case nothing has been proved...

We are told about lengthening our lifespan... extending our life... yet most people still die in their 50s or 60s when not younger...

Let's also remember that we have been keeping life records for just over 100 years for most of us... yet again go and visit cemeteries and you'll be surprise how long some of our forefathers live ! People who also lived healthy to their last day...

We are often told that this or that will kill us prematurely... yet half the people who take them lives to be very old !

Hungry for Diets

Everything you've always wanted to know about diets… and yet were never told !

Jesse CRAIGNOU

Everything works here as for cosmetics… we have nobody double to compare with… people can tells us whatever they like… as we don't have the first element of comparison… and we will never know !

Likewise we are forever told to eat more fruit and vegetable and never what we should eat more or less of… fruit and vegetables don't compose a diet !

One day as I was sitting to lunch with my friend Philip… he told me he had been on a diet and had lost 20 kilos…

I proceeded to congratulate him and ask him what diet he had been on… and he told me he had just 'eaten what he liked'… and '*What a wonderful diet !*' I thought to myself !

I realise again today that none of my pain has come to any gain… but the gut feeling that the answer is elsewhere… none of all those vigorous and valuable efforts had see the scale or my mind one way or the other… and yet the food I like suit me fine… and I would advise anyone asking me to go first and foremost for the food they like… as I'm sure we're closer to a solution there… and that would certainly limit the causes of our failures…

And after years of battles with all the many doctors I had seen… it was found that I was diabetic and needed daily insulin injections to balance my metabolism… no doctor had ever looked into that ! Goes to show that one should never lose hope !

#benefit, #cost, #diet, #disorder, #doctor, #eat, #food, #guide, #heal, #health, #junk, #nutrition, #recipe, #sport, #walk, #weight,

Jesse CRAIGNOU

At the end of the day… nothing, not one of all those diets, none of those products, none of those endeavours and efforts, none of those methods and approaches, none of those medicine, none of those deprivations, none of those talks, works ! And all that good money spent on medical research and patients over the years is wasted…

When we look a the food people eat in different cultures we see that there is statistically little difference between the Germans who eat a lot of fat foot and drink a lot of alcohol, the British who don't have lunch and eat a lot of sauces, drink a lot of alcohol and dine early, the Italians who eat a lot of starch and drink a lot of alcohol, and the French who have a very rich diet and drink a lot of alcohol… besides the Americans who often gather all the food aberrations…

Nature always has the last word… whatever we do… that' where its greatest strength lies and/or maybe its biggest shortcoming… and we're still hunting high and low for the diet that yield concrete positive results over the long run…

And if we often put weight on despite what we may eat… or don't eat… it is probably that it is in our nature… although we still need to refrain from overeating…

Nobody has the solution !

As to general practitioners, my doctor told me the other day : '*You know 20 mg or 40 mg… is virtually the same*'… and the chemist right behind him : '*19,5 mg or 21 mg is all the same !*'
The same people who will tell you to respect the prescribe dosage !
And you'd want me to believe them ?
Remember their good advice ? '*If in doubt ask your doctor*'… '*Your chemist your health expert*'…
Doctors are paid by the chemical industry to promote their medicine… and your chemist will sell you the medicine most profitable for him !

There are still and more and more overweight people in the world…
Does our body as greedy as it may for fat and sugar still run on the same fuel as our ancestors'… whereas it should have long adapted to the modern pace of life ?

Everyday we can read articles and studies… books even… promoting THE new diet that will write off all diets and turn overweight to history… and yet no sign of the slightest change… which should go to prove nobody has yet found the solution…

In studies shown on television in late 2014 we learn that exercise is not the solution to fitness, health and weight control…
Overweight and obese people may be in very good health… and slim people may suffer from a number of ailments normally blamed on overweight !

It is generally recognized that genetic make-up is the key to our weight whichever it may be and our health… any maybe even independently from one to the other… Germany has no problem exhibit these facts while France hides them…

#benefit, #cost, #diet, #disorder, #doctor, #eat, #food, #guide, #heal, #health, #junk, #nutrition, #recipe, #sport, #walk, #weight,

Jesse CRAIGNOU

Most people terrorise us by showing us only the fattest and most unhealthy... and for those who want to lose weight only remains the solution of plastic surgery...

Doctor Sharma left Germany to go and settle in Edmonton (Canada), and devised a new assessment of obesity... relevant to each patient taken individually... which he called the Obesity Staging System...

The obesity paradox shows the traditional relationship between health and weight is at best ludicrous...

In some cases the American National Cancer Institute even announces that moderate obesity may save lives in some diseases... which goes back to the case for cholesterol...

Dr Ingrid Mühlhauser (Hamburg) discovered the same thing in her studies...

Just as we had already noted that be slim does not necessarily promote health and longevity...

Achim Peters blames more stress than obesity... hence he developed the theory of the Selfish Brain...

If it only took changing, moderating, or modulating one's food and diet was the answer to overweight everybody would be slim ! As nobody likes to be overweight... not to mention the discomfort and extra cost of overweight...

Yet remains the question of the food industry in what goes on our plate... and more particularly when it comes to the content and the quality of our ingredients...

It seems, when we delve into the matter, that most people in the modern world in the 80s... curiously at a time when the food industry has taken over the control of food production... and has not stopped yet... earlier decades clearly exhibit a much slim figure... haven't we got food for thought here ? Research ? A topic that seems conspicuously avoided...

What are we really fed ?

Is there a recent food or ingredient or even element of food that the more sensitive people take in as overweight... without any other rhyme or reason... or still genetic reason whatsoever ?

And if there is indeed something there... why not simply withdraw it or reverse its effects for the better of mankind ?

In the 60s and 70s of my childhood and youth... virtually nobody was overweight... and the few that were overweight had to bear the cross of the ridicule others served them with every mean... too bad for them...

After that the trend for bodybuilding of the 80s... together with dance and gymnastics or keep fit... hid what was coming at a lot of us... who never saw what was coming at them !

Then everything seemed to change... the picture of the perfect body became blurred... the picture begins tear at the seams and crack...

#benefit, #cost, #diet, #disorder, #doctor, #eat, #food, #guide, #heal, #health, #junk, #nutrition, #recipe, #sport, #walk, #weight,

Jesse CRAIGNOU

We know that the chemicals, which come into play in the food industry present major risks and hazards… colourings and sweetener or taste enhancers… and what is used to substitute sugar and fat are often more noxious that sugar and fat… growth hormones… that even animals are -indirectly- farming or else… which come in to tamper with endocrines… such as antibiotics, which eventually end up in sewage water and dinking water… and are found as far as in mother's milk… all that via the natural recycling process !

The whole planet is completely polluted with all sorts of products… which end up in water, rainwater, rivers and seas and oceans… it's hardly worth what it takes to eat organic food… as genuine organic today is impossible to find on the planet… or only in extremely monitored conditions !

This may also explain why the Asian population, which remain undisturbedly slim…until they started eating non Asia food… at home or abroad… and the same goes for many populations in Africa… There is no two-ways about it… somebody has been playing with our food…

Nature managed to keep us slim and healthy… as long as we remained roaming and running in the original savannah to hunt and gather for our keep… but today… even if we exercise to exhaustion, the lack of exercise sees us reload our lost calories in our sedentary lives…

This brings us back to the old successful… eat everything within reason… and that's precisely what nutritionists advise us to do today… all tastes are found in nature… and some treatments may alter your sense of taste… such as chemotherapy… and eve change our staple diet… such as with insulin…

Statistics on life expectancy are pure speculation at best… a hoax at worst…
In fact today –and we all know a lot of them around us- a big fat number of people die around 50… and most of those deaths are not connected to illness or overweight…
The rest is only what laboratories want us to believe… so they can sell us their harmful chemicals… and intoxicate us further…
Many of our forefathers lived well beyond 50… the only difference being that a lot of them died –often along with their mothers- at birth or soon afterwards… for lack of hygiene (see Florence Nightingale's work on hygiene and how she probably saved mankind)…
We live barely longer than our forefathers in fact… many of us still die rather young of heart attacks for instance… they are neither old nor overweight for at least 50 – 75 % of them… nobody knows why nor how come… much to the loss of laboratories who lose good clients thereby…

#benefit, #cost, #diet, #disorder, #doctor, #eat, #food, #guide, #heal, #health, #junk, #nutrition, #recipe, #sport, #walk, #weight,

Jesse CRAIGNOU

Thank You

Thank you for buying my book…
I hope we have many more books to share together… making those moments even more highly valuable…

#benefit, #cost, #diet, #disorder, #doctor, #eat, #food, #guide, #heal, #health, #junk, #nutrition, #recipe, #sport, #walk, #weight,

page 78 of 87

Jesse CRAIGNOU

Words

Words have always been -and will always be- a major part of my life…

The moment I could read I read… and the moment I could write I wrote…
Words have always exercised that magic on me… and words more than anything or anyone have opened doors for me… more than anything or anyone could…

Words has a music of their own… Words will never let you down…

I write…
I write come what may…
I write whatever…
I write whenever…
I write wherever…
I write…

I wrote… before I could even write…

As soon as I put pen to paper, the first word is followed by another and another and another… and words tag on together… one after the other… and the words become my words for my greatest pleasure…
Words and I are words of a feather…

I look at my writing in more of an oral approach… spoken word's the written word here… our lips are not sealed…

My writing evolves around not only words and ideas but also reason and rhymes… sounds like poetry… imagine you're listening… and let yourself be carried away…
My words depict the surreal side of everyday life… with all its eerie magic… riding the crest of the jagged edge between fact and fiction…

The music of my words is my melody…

Play on words play with words… play on sounds play with sounds…

Adaptations, articles, books, lyrics, musicals, poetry, reviews, scenarios, short stories, songs, texts, …

#benefit, #cost, #diet, #disorder, #doctor, #eat, #food, #guide, #heal, #health, #junk, #nutrition, #recipe, #sport, #walk, #weight,

Hungry for Diets
Everything you've always wanted to know about diets… and yet were never told !

Jesse CRAIGNOU

Hungry for Diets is one of my books among which:

Pedagogical and business
- **Stories For English** (also an audiobook read by Tory L. WILSON)
- **Stories For English (Student's Edit)** (also an audiobook read by Dave WRIGHT)
- **Finger Licking Good (Student's Ed)** (also an audiobook read by Bobby BRIGHT)
- **Stories For English (Exercise And Practice)**
- **More Stories For English** (also an audiobook read by Kathy BRODERICK)
- **Stories For French**
- **Singin' To English**
- **The Comprehensive Teacher** (also an audiobook read by Maxine LENNON)
- **Business English Test**
- **Paris Passion**
- **Finger Licking Good**
- **Going Places**
- **Plain Sailing**
- **I Speak (A Little) English** (also an audiobook read by Jesse CRAIGNOU)
- **I Speak (A Little) French** (also an audiobook read by Jesse CRAIGNOU)

Books, eBooks and audiobooks
- **Live To Tell**
- **Righter** (also an audiobook read by Maxine LENNON)
- **BioHazard** (also an audio book read by David GEORGE)
- **A Woman's Day**
- **Booster Shot** (also an audio book read by David GEORGE)
- **Keeping Me Company** (also an audiobook read by Helen LLOYD)
- **In Between Stations**
- **Love Wars**
- **Hungry For Diets** (also an audiobook read by Jesse CRAIGNOU)
- **Ten A Penny**
- **Second Helpings**
- **Visionary Mountains** (also an audiobook read by Helen LLOYD)
- **Deflecting Patience**
- **Umma Dawn – The Confidential Files**
- **Redesigning Eden**
- **At The Gaytes Of Heaven**
- **Death Watch – A Matter Of Life**
- **Love… And Stuff Like That !**
- **To Think I Ran**
- **My Greatest Hits**
- **Poems & Songs**
- **Quilled ! Words Of A Feather**
- **Surrogate Life**
- **Danced A Little Tune**
- **Tales For Overgrown Children** (also an audiobook read by Jesse CRAIGNOU)

Children stories (with Franklin ERDER)
- **The Alison Eating Monster**

#benefit, #cost, #diet, #disorder, #doctor, #eat, #food, #guide, #heal, #health, #junk, #nutrition, #recipe, #sport, #walk, #weight,

Hungry for Diets
Everything you've always wanted to know about diets… and yet were never told !

Jesse CRAIGNOU

- **The Wolloes Have A Party** (also an audiobook read by Jesse CRAIGNOU)
- **The Wolloes Go To Bed**
- **The Little Stone Cutter**

#benefit, #cost, #diet, #disorder, #doctor, #eat, #food, #guide, #heal, #health, #junk, #nutrition, #recipe, #sport, #walk, #weight,

page 81 of 87

Hungry for Diets
Everything you've always wanted to know about diets… and yet were never told !

Jesse CRAIGNOU

Audio Books

Don't read much but ready to listen ?
Commuting ?

Try my audio books
Check Amazon, Audible & iTunes

Read by Bobby BRIGHT
• *Finger Licking Good*

Read by David GEORGE
• *BioHazard*
• *Booster Shot*

Read by Maxine LENNON
• *Righter*
• *The Comprehensive Teacher*

Read by Helen LLOYD
• *Keeping Me Company*
• *Visionary Mountains*

Read by Tory L. WILSON
• *Stories For English*

Read by Dave WRIGHT
• *Stories For English (Student's Edition)*

Read by Jesse CRAIGNOU
• *Tales For Overgrown Children*
• *Contes Pour Enfants Trop Grands*
• *I Speak (A Little) English*
• *I Speak (A Little) French*
• *To Think I Ran*
• *Histoires d'Iran*
• *Hungry For Diets*

Read by Kathy BRODERICK
• *More Stories For English*

Contact me: jesse.craignou@yahoo.fr

#benefit, #cost, #diet, #disorder, #doctor, #eat, #food, #guide, #heal, #health, #junk, #nutrition, #recipe, #sport, #walk, #weight,

Jesse CRAIGNOU

PodCasts

To further my work and give English teachers and students both a foreword and a top-up of what we can do together, I have created free PodCasts, which you can listen to again and again and download for free here :

For **English teachers and students**, *Stories for English* PodCast
http://www.podcasts.com/stories-for-english-dbef741c4

For **English Teachers** looking to further their teaching, *Desperate Teachers* PodCast
http://www.podcasts.com/desperate-teachers-a3f9804cb

For Desperate Slimmers, *Desperate Slimmers – Hungry for Diets* PodCast

For all those who like stories, French **teachers and students**, *Histoires* PodCast
http://www.podcasts.com/histoires-7a002ea0a

For more information and updates…
Contact me: jesse.craignou@yahoo.fr

#benefit, #cost, #diet, #disorder, #doctor, #eat, #food, #guide, #heal, #health, #junk, #nutrition, #recipe, #sport, #walk, #weight,

Hungry for Diets
Everything you've always wanted to know about diets… and yet were never told !

Jesse CRAIGNOU

Training & Coaching

I offer regular training and coaching sessions and workshops to professionals and individuals.

My services include training and coaching for
- Teachers and Trainers
- In-Company training
- Languages and Communication
- Writers and Authors
- The Media

I also translate from French into Italian, from French into English and back.

I train and coach on teaching and training in English, French, Italian, and Spanish.

My clients include top international businesses and professionals as well as top European managers (list on request).

#benefit, #cost, #diet, #disorder, #doctor, #eat, #food, #guide, #heal, #health, #junk, #nutrition, #recipe, #sport, #walk, #weight,

page 84 of 87

Hungry for Diets
Everything you've always wanted to know about diets… and yet were never told !

Jesse CRAIGNOU

Translating

I translate from French into Italian, from French into English… and back.

My services include training and coaching for
- Books
- Manuals and User's Guides
- Technical and Commercial documents
- Websites

For further information and feedback, to keep up with latest news, contact me:

jesse.craignou@yahoo.fr

More :
http://www.facebook.com/profile.php?id=716938953
or
http://www.viadeo.com/profile/0022elircedzsaht
or even
http://www.linkedin.com/profile/view?id=11065722&locale=en_US

My blogs :
http://paroles-et-musique.over-blog.com

My books and eBooks are on

kobo :
https://store.kobobooks.com/en-CA/search?query=Jesse%20CRAIGNOU&fcsearchfield=Author&fclanguages=all

YouScribe
http://www.youscribe.com/Search?quick_search=jesse+Craignou

Amazon:
http://www.amazon.com/s/ref=sr_nr_i_0?rh=k%3Ajesse+craignou%2Ci%3Astripbooks&keywords=jesse+craignou&ie=UTF8&qid=1370038010

SmashWords
https://www.smashwords.com/books/search?query=jesse+craignou

#benefit, #cost, #diet, #disorder, #doctor, #eat, #food, #guide, #heal, #health, #junk, #nutrition, #recipe, #sport, #walk, #weight,

Hungry for Diets
Everything you've always wanted to know about diets… and yet were never told !

Jesse CRAIGNOU

Looking to further you teaching ?

Singin' To English
http://en.youscribe.com/catalogue/educational-resources/art-music-and-cinema/music/singin-to-english-1533653

The Comprehensive Teacher
http://en.youscribe.com/catalogue/manuals-and-practical-information-sheets/education/languages/the-comprehensive-teacher-2003906
or
http://www.amazon.com/The-Comprehensive-Teacher/dp/B00I3PSDEO/ref=la_B00CMJY4HM_1_1?s=books&ie=UTF8&qid=1405533567&sr=1-1

Business English Test
http://en.youscribe.com/catalogue/educational-resources/education/teachers-resources/business-english-test-1914928

#benefit, #cost, #diet, #disorder, #doctor, #eat, #food, #guide, #heal, #health, #junk, #nutrition, #recipe, #sport, #walk, #weight,

Jesse CRAIGNOU

Paris Guide

Paris beauty… with your own private guide !

France is the number one destination for tourists in the world… and Paris is also the first tourist destination…
Visiting Paris is taking a walk through time and space… and the history of France, Europe and the world… offering a different style and facet of history and art turning every street corner…
Paris is also an industrious international business centre…

Whether you are visiting Paris for Business or pleasure, and wish to make more of its beauty and culture, contact **me at** <u>jesse.craignou@yahoo.fr</u> **for more information…**

#benefit, #cost, #diet, #disorder, #doctor, #eat, #food, #guide, #heal, #health, #junk, #nutrition, #recipe, #sport, #walk, #weight,

page 87 of 87